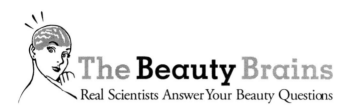

The **Beauty** Brains
Real Scientists Answer Your Beauty Questions

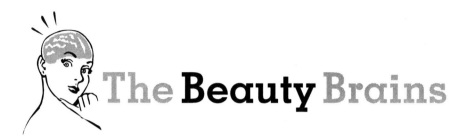

Real Scientists Answer Your Beauty Questions

edited by Sarah Bellum

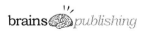

Brains Publishing – New York, Chicago

Published in the United States by Brains Publishing.
www.brainspublishing.com

ISBN: 978-0-9802173-4-6

Printed in the United States of America

First Edition

For Beauty Brainiacs everywhere ...

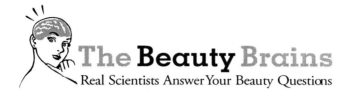

Table of Contents

Chapter 3
Hair Myths

Section II Skin

Chapter 4
Skin Treatments – From Silly to Sublime

Chapter 5
Beauty Biology

Section III Makeup

Chapter 6
Marvelous Makeup

Chapter 7
Nail Knowledge You Need

Chapter 8
The Science of Smell

Section IV Beauty Industry

Chapter 9
Scandals and Secrets of the Beauty Biz

Chapter 10
Cosmetic Surgery

Chapter 11
Cosmetic Concerns & Perilous Products

Appendix

Who are the Beauty Brains?

The Beauty Brains are a group of cosmetic scientists who understand what the chemicals used in cosmetics really do, how products are tested, and what all the advertising means. They have no cosmetics to sell so you can be sure that the information provided is the most unbiased beauty advice available.

Left Brain

The most hardcore skeptical scientist of all the Beauty Brains, the Left Brain peruses the world of science to bring you the latest developments and how they might apply to the cosmetic world.

Right Brain

Still scientific, but a bit less militant, the Right Brain has a good eye for the humorous, and human interest, side of science. The Right is particularly skilled in interpreting advertising claims.

Sarah Bellum

The more sensitive Beauty Brain, Sarah focuses on the aesthetics of the cosmetic world and is more likely to find stories on the pages of People than Pubmed.

The Other Lobes

The other Brains work behind the scenes researching questions, reviewing the latest beauty technology, and keeping up with the day to day business of running this website. As we continue to grow, you'll be hearing from some of the other "lobes." All of us use "brainy" nicknames because being anonymous lets us blog about all kinds of products from many different companies without any bias.

What's the Purpose of The Beauty Brains?

There are literally THOUSANDS of cosmetic products constantly bombarding you with confusing and sometimes, false information. The Beauty Brains was started in 2006 to help women understand the real science behind the beauty products they use everyday. We have taken questions from people around the world about all beauty topics including hair care, skin care, make up and even cosmetic surgery.

We're here to help you cut through the confusing, misleading and sometimes false information that the beauty companies bombard you with. Our goal is to explain cosmetic science to you in a way that's entertaining and easy to understand. We believe the more information you have, the better you'll be able to find products that you like at a price you can afford. So, you can listen to the advertising. Or advice from a friend. Or what your stylist tells you. But if you want to really understand cosmetic products in an unbiased, scientific way.

In this book we've collected more than 100 of our best questions and answers to make learning about cosmetic science easy and entertaining. By giving you honest, unbiased information, The Beauty Brains can help you become a smarter shopper so you'll be able to get the products you like at prices you can afford.

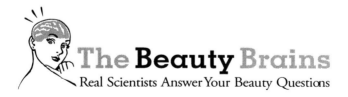

The **Beauty** Brains
Real Scientists Answer Your Beauty Questions

Chapter 1
Hair Products and How They Work

The Shampoo Secret Beauty Companies Don't Want You To Know

Conny tells The Beauty Brains she has a very sensitive scalp with fine hair and suffers from hair loss and dandruff. Dermatologists have advised her to use a clear gel shampoo that has to be clarifying or deep cleansing. So, she's tried Suave Daily Clarifying Shampoo, Suave for Men Deep Cleansing shampoo, Neutrogena Anti-residue shampoo, and Prell Classic original formula. She's not happy with those choices and is asking us to set her straight.

The Right Brain responds:

While we hate to disagree with dermatologists, we don't understand why they recommended a deep cleansing shampoo when you have dandruff. Deep cleansing type shampoos will remove the surface flakes, but only a dandruff shampoo can control the cause of flaking and itching. So we'd recommend finding a good dandruff shampoo instead of chasing deep cleaning, clarifying and anti-residue products. This may seem confusing to you because the beauty companies tell you there are SO many different kinds of shampoo. But in reality, every shampoo on the market falls into a few basic categories.

Only 4 different shampoo types in the world

All shampoo can be categorized by their basic functional category. So then why are there eleventy million products on the market, you ask? Because the companies that sell shampoo need to find new ways to talk about their products to keep them sounding new and exciting. There's nothing wrong with them being creative about their names and claims as long as the companies are honestly depicting what their products can do. But you can be a smarter consumer if you can see beyond the marketing hype and understand the functionality of these 4 basic shampoo types.

1. Deep Cleansing Shampoos (Also known as Volumizing, Clarifying, Balancing, Oil Control, and Thickening.) These shampoos are designed to get gunk off your hair and scalp. They typically contain slightly higher levels of detergents so they foam and clean better. They include the examples above as well as salon products like Paul Mitchell Shampoo 2. and Frederic Fekkai's Full Volume.

2. Conditioning Shampoos (Aka Moisturizing, 2 in 1, Smoothing, Anti-frizz, Strengthening, Color Care, Straightening, and Hydrating) This kind of formula is all about leaving a moisturizing agent, like a silicone or Polyquaternium 10, on the hair to smooth it. It's very good for dry hair, especially if you color treat or heat style but it can weigh down fine hair. Good examples of this type includes most of the Pantene formulas and some products from the L'Oreal Vive collection and Dove ProCare.

3. Baby Shampoos (Aka Kids shampoo, and Tear-free)
Johnson's Baby Shampoo is the classic example but this category also includes Touch Of An Angel and The Little Bath. These are milder, lower foaming surfactant formulas that are designed not to sting or burn your eyes. They're better for babies but they don't clean hair as well.

4. Anti-Dandruff Shampoos (Aka Anti-itch, Flake Control, and Dry Scalp)
Head and Shoulders is the leading dandruff product; other examples include Nizoral and Redken Dandruff Control . These are medicated shampoos that contain a drug ingredient that controls itching and flaking. In the United States these are considered to be Over-the-Counter (OTC) Drugs.

The Beauty Brains bottom line

Hopefully, this helps you better understand the marketing hype around shampoo names. We're not saying that all shampoos are the same, or even that all shampoos in a given category type are the same. There are real performance differences so it's important that you shop around and find a product that performs the way you like at a price that you can afford. But just don't get too hung up on the names the companies use to describe the products. That's the marketing part of the industry, not the science part.

Is Paul Mitchell Making Your Hair Break?

Jackie's question:
About a year ago my stylist starting using Paul Mitchell products on me and I haven't loved my hair since! Now it's damaged and it breaks easily. My stylist blames me using the flat iron. I know that doesn't help BUT I used the flat iron for years and have never had this happen. She tells me that's because I had my hair colored so much. I have never had these problems until she switched to Paul Mitchell. Is it possible that his products make my hair start to break off and thin out?

The Left Brain's snappy comment:

Jackie, thanks so much for the question. I see how you could think that Paul Mitchell made your hair go bad, but I doubt that's really what happened. Paul Mitchell products are not different enough from other products you've been using (except for being overpriced), so there is likely a different reason you're experiencing hair breakage. It is natural to leap to conclusions like this, but they are often incorrect.

Instead of worrying about Paul Mitchell, I'd blame 3 other factors for your hair problem:

  1. Flat iron usage is VERY bad for your hair. That's probably the most immediate cause of daily breakage. If you want less damage consider ironing less frequently.

  2. In the long run, the worst thing you can is chemically color your hair. Coloring breaks down the hair's protein making it weaker. Frequent chemical processing literally pushes your hair to its "breaking point."

  3. The first two factors are worsened because you're getting older and your hair is weaker. As we age our hair gets less dense and more prone to breakage. That's probably why you're seeing so much hair breakage more recently - Father Time is catching up with you!

What to do

So, what can you do? Well, the shampoo doesn't matter much as long as you're using a conditioner. The Paul Mitchell conditioner is good, but so are many other cheaper, mass market brands like Fructis, Pantene, or Tresemme. You might consider using one of these every time you do your hair. The conditioner should provide enough lubrication so that pulling on it with a comb does not break the hair. It may even provide some protection against the heat of the flat iron. If you're not using a conditioner, be sure to use a conditioning shampoo like Pantene 2-in-1. This should help slow your hair breaking problem.

The Beauty Brains bottom line:
In truth, heat, coloring, and age are all conspiring against you to break your hair. You can't do anything about the aging process but if you stopped coloring and reduced the heat exposure, your hair would break less. Of course, then you might not like how it looks. Such is the price we pay for beauty!

Is Ojon Restorative Treatment Any Good?

Anonymous Asks:
I was curious about what you thought of the Ojon products, specifically their restorative hair treatment. Is this any better than other products, and how would it work to improve your hair?

The Right Brain Responds:
Ojon's oil treatment consists of palm oil, fragrance, and a few extracts. It's particularly interesting because recent research has shown that only SOME oils will actually penetrate the hair. Mineral oil and sunflower oil, for example, will not penetrate. But coconut oil (which is essentially the same as palm oil) will filter deep into the cortex because it is so similar to hair's natural lipids.

Oil conditions hair
Why is that a big deal? Because the natural oils in your hair help make it flexible and waterproof. Washing your hair removes some of these natural oils. So it is possible that applying coconut oil to your hair can fight some of the effects of this oil loss. Once inside the hair, the oil serves as a re-fatting agent. However, this type of conditioning won't have much effect on the cuticle, the outer layer of hair, so you'll still need to use a good conditioner to smooth the hair and make it easier to comb.

Is it a good value? Well, that's another question. Any other coconut oil based product should do about the same job and should be much cheaper. Off hand we can't recommend any specific brands, but look for products that feature coconut oil as the first ingredient. (If anyone has any recommendations we'd be glad to review them. Just let us know.)

Is there anything to their rain forest hype? Well, their rain forest story seems well intentioned but this ingredient isn't proven to work any better or any differently than non-rain forest ingredients. Coconut trees only grow in tropical climates, but there's nothing special about trees from the rain forest. So, if you like Ojon's products and you want to support their cause AND you can afford the $55 for this product, then by all means buy it. But don't buy the product just because they tell you their rain forest extract is better.

The Beauty Brains Bottom Line

We haven't tested this product but based on recent scientific research, the palm oil used by Ojon should penetrate the hair. Therefore it could protect your hair from over-washing. However, at $55, it's a bit pricey so shop around for other coconut oil products because you may be able to get the same effect for less money.

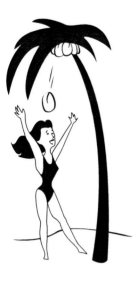

Two Natural Oils That Make Your Hair Shiny and Strong

Lina says:

I was very happy to read your post about coconut oil penetrating hair. I have been using it for a while and feel my hair is stronger than it used to be. I'd like to keep using coconut oil and I want to add olive oil to make my hair shiny but I'm worried that mixing the two oils will stop the coconut oil from penetrating. Is it ok to mix two oils on my hair? Thanks for all of your helpful information - you've kept me from wasting money on over-hyped products.

The Left Brain provides an oily update:

Thanks for your kind words, Lina. Yes, studies have shown that coconut oil actually penetrates the hair to help make it stronger. And as it turns out, olive oil also has penetrating properties. Scientists at the Textile Research (*J. Cosmet.Sci 52, 169-184, 2001*) tested Olive oil, Avocado oil, Meadow foam seed oil, Sunflower oil, and Jojoba oil. Their results showed that straight chain glycerides like olive oil easily penetrate into the hair. Polyunsaturated oils, like Jojoba oil, are more open in their structure so they don't pass through the layers of cuticles very well.

What does that mean in plain English? Olive and Avocado oils penetrate all the way into the hair shaft. Meadowfoam seed oil partially penetrates, and jojoba and sunflower oils don't penetrate at all. They're very superficial and don't really provide any practical benefit. Kind of like Ryan Seacrest.

And to answer your question:

Mixing coconut and olive oils shouldn't be a problem. In fact, it's possible that the olive/coconut oil combination might even penetrate hair better. I won't bore you with the details, but it has to do with mixed micelles. I'd start with a 50/50 mixture and see how that works for your hair.

Is Pantene Good Or Bad For My Hair?

Sophie Says:

I've heard a lot of things about Pantene Pro-V's shampoo and conditioners. A lot of hairstylists swear on their hair-dryers that it is awful for your hair. Supposedly, it coats your hair with plastic or wax to make it seem smooth, soft, and shiny, instead of really moisturizing your hair. It also reportedly makes your scalp itchy and hair fall out.

However, I've been using the Pantene Restoratives shampoo and conditioner for a few months now, and I find my hair less frizzy, more manageable, smoother, and softer. Of course, I also use John Frieda Anti-Frizz Serum and Pantene Pro-V Restoratives Frizz Control Ultra Smoothing Balm (I highly recommend the latter, just apply to wet hair). Phew, that was long. So, my question is: Is Pantene good or bad for my hair?

The Right Brain Righteously Responds:

Sophie, please don't fall into the trap of believing everything your stylist tells you. (That's one of the The Beauty Brains Basic Beliefs.) While most stylists are very talented at cutting and styling hair, they're not very talented at interpreting cosmetic formulations.

The truth is, Pantene's shampoo and conditioner formulas are believed to be among the best in the industry by those of us in the cosmetic science side of the business. It makes sense if you think about it. P&G, makers of Pantene, have a HUGE research budget. Certainly larger than any salon company. That means they can afford to dedicate resources to developing and testing the best formulas possible. We've seen Pantene formulas beat the pants of salon products in blind consumer testing. (The products are hidden or blinded, not the consumers)

Why is Pantene vilified?

So why do stylists say that Pantene coats the hair with plastic, or make it fall out? Because that's what they're told by the sales representatives for the salon companies. And the truth is, it's just not true! Compare the ingredient lists for Pantene conditioner and any salon brand you can find.

Even though the names vary you'll see three basic types of ingredients: fatty alcohols (like cetyl and stearyl alcohol); conditioning ingredients (like stearamidopropylamine and quaternium-18) and silicones (like dimethicone and cyclomethicone.) There's nary a plastic to be found in Pantene. And no, it doesn't make your hair fall out either.

The Beauty Brains bottom line
You can choose whatever you like - a retail brand like Pantene or a salon brand like Matrix. But shop around and find a product you like and make your own decisions based on your own experience. Don't pass on Pantene because of stylist anti-hype.

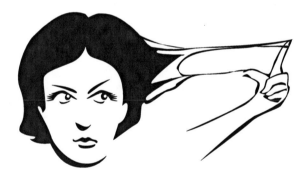

Are salon products in regular stores the same as those in salons

One reader wanted to know if the salon products that you buy at the local Kroger (general store) are the same as the ones you can buy at a salon. The answer referenced a story by a news team out of Fort Meyers, Florida. The story was so biased and misinformed we thought a balanced, Beauty Brains insider response was needed.

The idea that salon products are different than store ones is interesting. We are cosmetic chemists that work in the industry and know that this story is a bit skewed. If the news reporters wanted to get the "real" story, they shouldn't be asking the head of Paul Mitchell because he is completely biased. They should ask chemists that make products.

Discovering Diversion
The truth is these salon brands depend on 'diverted' product to boost their sales. They want to have it both ways. They want to tell you that Paul Mitchell is a salon-only brand which makes it seem more exclusive, but they also want the high volume sales that they can only get through mass market outlets like your local Kroger. Additionally, they don't want to anger their salon distributors because people are able to get the same stuff but for cheaper.

They make up this story of products being inferior. In nearly all cases, they are not. The way diversion works is this. Paul Mitchell hires a company to manufacture their products. Then Paul Mitchell sales people get and fill orders from distributors. Distributors are legitimate businesses that sell directly to independent salons. The distributors can order as much as they want, then sell it to the salons who can then sell it to you.

Follow the money
Some of these distributors work directly with stores like Kroger, Albertsons, etc. So when these stores put in an order (a really big order compared to a salon) the distributors just order more product from Paul Mitchell to fill the Kroger order.

Paul Mitchell doesn't even question the big orders because they like the extra sales. They turn a blind eye to what's going on just so they can express public "outrage" that their product is being sold at the local drugstore. This is bunch of bunk.

The stuff you get at the local Kroger is every bit as good as the stuff you get at the salon. Don't be fooled. If the folks at Paul Mitchell really wanted to stop these sales, they would simply question their distributors and find out who is selling to Kroger, or Target or Albertson.

The problem of counterfeiting is a real one, but it's not something that you'll find at large stores like Kroger. That company is not going to sell something contaminated because they would be sued in a heartbeat. The places that are a little more sketchy are the small shops (some salons) with the dust on top of the bottles. Those are the places you have to worry about.

The Beauty Brains bottom line
You can trust that if you're buying a salon brand from a regular store, there is no difference between it and the stuff you can get at a salon.

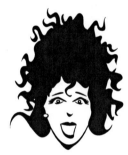

Do Curling Shampoos Really Work?

Charlotte Comments:
I'd love to believe that those curling shampoos will really shape my thick hair. What do the Brain's Believe?

The Right Brain Responds:
Well, Charlotte, this is an easy one. Curling shampoos do NOT make your hair curly. In fact, if you read the labels carefully, some of them don't even SAY they'll make your hair curly!

Examine the bottle
Let's take a look, shall we? Even the most flagrant offender of the truth, Wash n' Curl shampoo, only IMPLIES that it will make your hair curly just from shampooing. Read the label carefully - it says it provides "the most beautiful curls with body, bounce and resilience after styling." Well, duh! If the shampoo only makes your hair curly AFTER you style it, it's not really doing much for you is it?

What else does Wash n' Curl say? "Your hair will be extremely curl responsive … Even dry, damaged, color treated hair will have the staying power of thick curly hair… Its special Curl Enhancers infuse hair with the Holding Power of naturally curly hair."

The only piece of truth in this claim is that the shampoo does contain something that could be called a "curl enhancer." Looking at the ingredient list we see that it does contains a polymer (Acrylates/C10-30 Alkyl Acrylate Crosspolymer), that COULD provide some styling benefits. But that would only work if it wasn't rinsed out!

Remember, just because a product contains an ingredient that does something, it doesn't mean that it does something in that product!

The rest of the claims are pretty much made up, as far as we can tell. There is no shampoo technology that will measurably improve the holding power of your hair.

Other curling shampoos
What about other products, you ask? Well here's two more:

KMS Curl Up Shampoo and Marc Anthony Strictly Curls. Neither of these shampoos make strong curling claims. KMS only promises to be your "curl's best friend, " to " start your style in the shower," and to "boost boisterous curls while adding moisture and shine."

Marc, on the other hand, offers to protect color; repair dry, frizzy areas, and repel humidity to define shiny, soft, curls. ("Define" curls is not really a very emphatic claim.) Aside from a little polyquaternium (a conditioning ingredient) neither of these products have any curling technology either.

We could go on and on, but you get the picture. These shampoos don't have anything in them to make your hair curly. They don't even really do anything to prepare your hair for styling, other than getting it clean.

The Beauty Brains bottom line

If you really want curly hair, go buy some mousse. Or, God forbid, get a perm!

Chapter 2
Tips on Caring for Your Hair

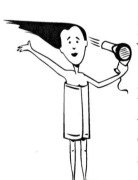

Drying Dilemma:
What's The Best Way To Dry Your Hair?

Ellie asks:
I usually don't have the patience to blow dry my hair completely. But my hair dresser told me it is better to dry the hair roots completely than half blow drying the hair and then let it dry by itself. Is it true?

The Right Brain responds:
We think this idea is kind of silly but we'll avoid the temptation to just tell you to get a new hair dresser and instead we'll try to present both sides of the story.

Technically Speaking
It's more damaging to blow dry or towel dry your hair than it is to let it air dry. It's as simple as that. That's because heat from blow dryers can mess with the natural lipid distribution in your hair AND degrade the intercellular cement that holds the hair's protective cuticle in place. And the physical abrasion from towel drying not only loosens healthy cuticles but can actually wear them away! So if you dry your hair a lot you'll end up with less shine and more split ends.

Stylistically Speaking
We assume a hair dresser would argue that blow drying keeps your hair sleek and smooth and that air drying makes it frizzy. At least this is what the hairdressers we have worked with think.

So, Ellie, it looks like the answer to your drying dilemma could come down to what's more important to you: avoiding damage or fighting frizz? Less damage is better for your long term hair health but nobody wants frizz. Only you can decide which to choose. But, hey, if you're THAT worried about frizz you can always use a good smoothing product after you dry your hair. You can buy an entire CASE of this effective frizz fighter for only 20 bucks!

3 Simple Secrets To Save Your Scalp

Ebesan says:

I'm a male who's very happy with my baldness I don't want new hair. But, I do want my scalp to look better. It's blotchy and discolored with different layers of skin. Is there a product, or procedure that can give me back my healthy scalp skin?

The Right Brain Responds:

Hi Eb, we're always glad to answer questions from our male readers! Without actually examining your scalp it's hard to say what's going on upstairs, but here are 3 tips that might help:

1. Suds your skull

What are you washing your scalp with? Bar soap? That might be stripping your skin of essential oils. Try baby shampoo or a mild body wash.

2. Chrome your dome

Are you applying sunscreen to your head? You should! Even if you wear a hat most of the time you might be getting enough UV radiation to damage your skin. What? You're a guy and you don't know anything about girly things like sunscreen??? Get over it and start using sunscreen. Your hair will thank you.

3. Soothe your scalp

If your skin is blotchy and scaly, you might try a hydrocortizone cream to see if that calms it down.

If none of these ideas help, we'd recommend seeing a dermatologist. Visits to these doctors are almost always worth it.

Want Shiny Hair? Avoid The Dulling Dozen!

Tammy's turmoil:
Can you tell me what makes hair really shiny?

The Right Brain's shimmering reply:
Naturally shiny hair has a cuticle that's smooth and flat; it's plumped up with water (about 10 to 15% by weight); and it's rich in natural oils that keep the whole thing "glued" together.

Unfortunately, you're stealing shine from your hair everyday and you probably don't even realize it. If you want good gloss, you should avoid these 12 things that can rob hair of shine. Or as we like to call them, the Dulling Dozen:

1. Flood Damage
Even "harmless" water can be a shine stealer. That's because too much moisture swells the hair shaft and causes the cuticle to buckle. The more frequently you wet your hair, the less shine you're likely to have.

2. Shampoo Scrubbing
Scrubbing bubbles seem cute but all that rub a dub dub lifts the cuticle even more. Using a conditioning shampoo can help because the hair shafts won't snag against each other when you're lathering up.

3. Careless Under-conditioning
Ok, not everyone needs to condition EVERY time they wash their hair. BUT, if your hair is dry to begin with it's much more likely to be damaged during and after styling if you skip conditioner. You're just giving shine away!

4. Death by Towel Drying
So, now your hair is wet. What do you do? Blot, don't rub! A rough towel can cause an amazing amount of damage on wet hair.

5. The Brush Off
Don't fall for that old myth that you should brush you hair 100 strokes every night. While brushing does temporarily help by distributing natural oils, in the long run it strips off layers of cuticle and weakens hair.

6. Hot Styling Appliances
Heat is the natural enemy of shine. That's because high temperatures damage the natural lipids (fancy word for oils) that help keep hair flexible and shiny. If you do decide to heat style, use protection!

7. Protective Product Residue

Yes, you do need to use heat protection but be careful what you wish for. Some leave in creams and gels leave behind a dulling residue.

8. Color My World

Chemical coloring is very damaging because it breaks down the inner structure of hair protein. Even if you use the special conditioner that comes with the coloring kit, your hair never fully recovers.

9. Wave Bye Bye

Permanent waving is another chemical process that's highly damaging.

10. Twist and Shout

Twisting and playing with your hair is a dangerous habit as far as shine is concerned. That's because the torsional forces (fancy word for twisting and bending) loosens the cuticles.

11. I Dig A Pony

Wearing your hair in a pony tail may seem like a hassle free style, but if you pull it back too tightly you may be creating micro-fractures in the hair that will reflect light unevenly and cause loss of shine.

12. Here Comes The Sun

And with the sun comes damaging UV radiation that can wreak havoc on natural hair lipids like 18-methyleicosinoic acid. Without these lipids hair dulls quickly. If you can't stay out of the sun make sure you're protecting your hair with a good conditioner.

How To Tell If A Dandruff Shampoo Will Really Work

Maaiki Is Feeling Flakey:
I was wondering what your opinion is of Burt's Bees Feelin' Flaky shampoo. Looking over the ingredients list, it looks like they did a good job of avoiding skin irritants (except for the tea tree oil), but since it all gets washed off after a few seconds, I don't know how much good it could do. The ingredients are, Vegetable glycerin, lemon fruit water, sucrose cocoate, decyl polyglucose, willowbark extract, peppermint leaf extract (organic), willow leaf extract, burdock root extract, nettles leaf extract, yucca schidigera extract, cedar leaf oil, tea tree oil, lemon oil, rosemary oil, juniper oil, peppermint oil, xanthan gum (natural thickener), glucose & glucose oxidase & lactoperoxidase.

The Left Brain Gets Indignant:
You've discovered one of the shampoo scams that REALLY makes The Beauty Brains mad - false and misleading anti-dandruff claims. Some companies make it APPEAR that their products will control dandruff but they really won't. The way companies do this may not be strictly illegal, but it certainly is unethical in my opinion. Let's look at this Burt's Bees product as an example.

Burt's Bees Feeling Flaky Shampoo
According to Drugstore.com, the full name of the product is Burt's Bees Doctor Burt's Herbal Treatment Shampoo with Cedar Leaf & Juniper Oil. Doctor Burt, huh? I know that the reference is tongue-in-cheek, but that sure sounds medicinal to me! Strike One.

Below the name it describes the shampoo as Feelin' Flaky? with a question mark. In the context of cleaning hair and scalp, "flaky" is generally the term used to describe a symptom of dandruff. (Itchiness is another symptom.) Hmmm. Strike Two.

And finally the use directions: Wet hair, lather, rinse, then lather and rinse again. Shampoo at least three times a week for maximum effectiveness."

Maximum effectiveness? Again, sounds like they're promising some kind of sustained effect. If they're not talking about dandruff, what effectiveness are they talking about? Just getting your hair clean. That's lame - Strike 3!

While this product, and others like it, don't overtly claim to control dandruff, they are CERTAINLY making that implication. And that's the same as lying to consumers.

What's In A Real Dandruff Shampoo

The truth is, dandruff shampoos contain active ingredients that treat the physiological causes of dandruff. How can you tell if a shampoo is really effective against dandruff? In the US, look for active drug ingredients like Zinc Pyrithione (also known as ZPT.) In Europe and a few other countries, look for Octopyrox on the label. If you don't see some kind of legitimate active ingredient listed it's not really an effective dandruff shampoo. Don't believe everything the cosmetic companies tell you!

The Beauty Brains bottom line

You ask "how much good" this product will do for you. Well, it will certainly get your hair clean. The primary surfactants (sucrose cocoate and decyl polyglucose) will see to that. And it won't dry your scalp out either, those are pretty mild cleansers. But that's about it. It's not a medicated shampoo so it won't help against dandruff.

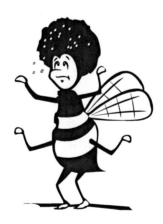

You Don't Have To Use Body Wash To Get Yourself Clean

Valeri is vexed:
Body wash can cost $4 or more. Some shampoos cost .66 to .99 cents. Is there that much of a difference between the two products to justify the price? I use the shampoo for body wash.

Left Brain's bubbly reply:
Great question Valeri and an astute observation for even considering the possibility. The truth is that shampoos and body washes are so similar that they can be used interchangeably. In fact, in the early days of body washes it was not uncommon for a company to take its shampoo formula, put it in a different bottle, change the label and call it a body wash.

Shampoo & Body Wash Similarities
Let's look at some of the things that the two products have in common.

1. Water & detergent. Shampoos and body washes are designed to clean which means they're mostly water and detergent. And for cleaning oil off of surfaces nothing beats surfactants. Body washes like Dove, Olay and Herbalessences all use Sodium Laureth Sulfate. This is the same surfactant that many shampoos use.

2. Fragrance & Color. No differences here. Body wash and shampoo use the same ingredients to make the product smell good and look pretty.

3. Conditioning ingredients. Since detergents can be a bit harsh, ingredients are added to improve the after-feel of hair and skin. Often body washes and shampoos use the same types of ingredients.

Shampoo & Body Wash Differences
While shampoos and body washes are quite similar there are some important differences.

1. Body wash uses less harsh detergents. Since skin is generally more sensitive than hair, body wash formulas are made with slightly less detergent and also less harsh detergents. The low cost shampoos use SLS or ALS which are excellent cleaners but can be drying to skin.

2. Different conditioning ingredients. Some of the ingredients that conditioner hair can also provide a nice feel on skin. However, many will not and this is often a key difference between shampoos & body washes.

A great comparison is to look at the list of ingredients of the Herbal Essences Body Wash versus their Shampoo. See the similar ingredients?

Companies have actually picked up on the similarities. In the Old Spice High Endurance Body Wash they show a guy washing his hair and body with the same product.

The Beauty Brains bottom line
Shampoos clean and so do body washes. In general you'll find it beneficial to use both a body wash and a shampoo. But there is really no reason you couldn't use a shampoo to clean your entire body. If you use a daily moisturizer, then there is no need for a separate body wash.

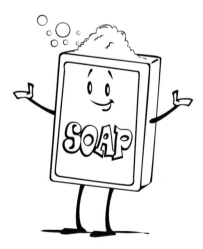

Top 10 Split End Busters

One of our fave forums for hair facts is The Long Hair Forum. If you want to grow your hair longer, it is THE site to see. They have put together a great list of tips. Here are the top 10 that will actually help improve your hair. You can also read their original list "Keeping Splits At Bay: Secrets of Gently Handling Your Hair"*

1. Move your mane
If your hair is long enough to get caught under coat collars or under shoulder straps (for Messenger bags, back pack, etc) then be sure to move your hair before putting on that bag.

2. Keep air off your hair
Does your hair whip in the wind? Wind knots up hair. Knots damage length. Damaged length causes more splits. Eventually the damaged length splits. Restrain your hair when you are going to be in a lot of wind.

3. Wash warily
Only apply shampoo to roots where it needs it. Avoid washing the dried out ends.

4. Be picky about piling hair on top
Do you pile your hair on top of your head when you shampoo? This creates MANY opportunities for splits. Shampoo really only needs to be applied to your roots. That's where the grease/oil is. Personally, I condition the length of my hair, apply shampoo to my scalp (down to ears), rinse, then apply conditioner again, rinse. This is called CWC (Condition Wash Condition). All the while, the length of my hair just hangs down my back.

5. Towel drying is treacherous
When you dry your hair, do you scrub your scalp with a towel? It feels great, but it will rip, strip, pop, snap and fry your hair in no time! Many of us use some sort of a turbie type towel/turban for drying our hair. Others put a towel on their back and let the hair drip onto the towel.

6. Blow off blow drying
Do you blow dry your hair? The heat and the wind created by the blowfryer (no that isn't a typo) really damages hair, too. Any heat styling tool can potentially damage hair. If you feel you must use them, keep the temperature low and exposure time to your hair short.

*http://forums.longhaircommunity.com/showthread.php?t=5816%20%5B/URL

7. Subdue your shampoo

How often do you shampoo? Regardless of HOW you shampoo, how OFTEN do you do it? Many of us have found that 2-3 shampooings per week is sufficient. It takes a few weeks to train your scalp to have fewer washings, but it helps protect the ends. Not everyone has success with fewer shampooings, though.

8. Condition, condition, condition

Do you use conditioner or a cream rinse when you shampoo? My personal belief is, if you want long hair you need to condition it EVERY time you shampoo. If nothing else, it helps detangle my hair. You also might consider using a leave in conditioner, especially one that helps detangle (and gives slip).

9. Oil often

You can oil the length of your hair daily. Many long hairs do this. They put a small drop in the palm of their hand, rub their hands together and lightly apply the oil to the ends only of the hair. There is an abundance of oils that you can use, some are quite exotic. Extra virgin olive oil (EVOO) is probably the most common, but there is a long list of oils everyone has tried and ones that each person likes/doesn't like.

10. Consider combing cautiously

After you've shampooed, when/how do you brush/comb your hair? Generally, brushing wet hair is bad for the hair. Hair is most delicate when wet. Brushing tends to stretch the strands. Stretching the strands puts wear and tear, which causes damage, which causes splits.

How To Clean Your Hair With Conditioner

Nina needs to know...

about WEN, a line of cleansing conditioners created by a Hollywood hair stylist Chaz Dean. Dean believes that sulfates in most shampoos can be very damaging and stripping to hair so he created these cleansing conditioners to clean hair without stripping it. Nina wants to know if hair can really be better off in the long run by cleansing with a conditioner. And if it does work, will a regular drugstore conditioner produce the same effect.

The Left Brain replies:

Great question, Nina. First of all, the idea of cleaning your hair with conditioner is not new and was not invented by Chaz. And no, he's not using any kind of revolutionary technology. Let's take a look at the ingredients:

Water, glycerin, cetyl alcohol, rosemary leaf extract, wild cherry fruit extract, fig extract, chamomile extract, marigold flower extract, behentrimonium methosulfate, cetearyl alcohol, stearamidopropyl dimethylamine, amodimethicone, hydrolized wheat protein, polysorbate 60, panthenol, menthol, sweet almond oil, PEG-60 almond glycerides, methylisothiazolinone, methylchloroisothiazolinone, citric acid, essential oils.

Looking at just the functional ingredients (leaving out extracts, preservatives, pH adjusters,) leaves the following:

glycerin, cetyl alcohol, behentrimonium methosulfate, cetearyl alcohol, stearamidopropyl dimethylamine (SADMA), and amodimethicone

Common conditioner

These are very common conditioner ingredients. Here's what they do: Glycerin can provide moisturization in a leave on product, but it doesn't do anything for hair when it's rinsed out. Cetyl and cetearyl alcohol are thickening and emulsifying agents are are used to make a conditioner rich and creamy. Because they're oil soluble they could, in theory, help lift some of the sebum of your hair and scalp. Behentrimonium methosulfate, SADMA, and amodimethicone are very effective conditioning ingredients because they deposit on the hair.

Could you clean your hair with this product? Sure, if your hair isn't very dirty this could work pretty well. But so could any basic conditioner. In fact, I'd look for a conditioner that doesn't have any silicone in it, just to make sure it leaves as little on your hair as possible.

But what if you have greasy hair, or if you use hairspray, mousse gel, or putty? Then cleansing conditioners are not a very good idea. They don't have enough cleansing power to remove gunk from the hair. Chances are that cleansing with conditioner will leave your hair feeling dirty and weighed down.

The Beauty Brains bottom line:
If you're really worried about drying your hair out from over-shampooing, there's nothing wrong with skipping your shampoo and just rinsing with conditioner once in a while. But you don't need to spend $28 on a special product. A nice inexpensive drug store brand will do the same thing.

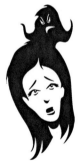

Hair Extensions May Be Killing Your Hair

Today's question comes from Heather whose experiment with professional hair extensions turned into a nightmare.

Heather writes:
I got hair extensions out almost two years ago. I paid four thousand dollars for the kind that are put on individually with clips, which need to be put in and taken out with a tool that only salons have they have to be adjusted every month.

After about nine months, as the stylist was adjusting the clips, I noticed that my hair was coming out along with the extensions! There just was no more hair below the clip of hair extension hair. My hair was just GONE. It all broke off at hundreds of different places where the clips were attached. It looked like a horror film!

I cried for months. Now my hair is still growing from my roots, but it's not getting longer. Is there anything I can do to help strengthen my hair and stop it from breaking? If I were a multi-millionaire, would there be some way? Do movie stars have some way they repair their hair we don't know about?

The Brains Respond:
Heather, your story is really touching and we're so sorry for what you've gone through. Based on your description, you have a condition known as Traction Alopecia a type of hair loss that is caused by pulling on hair. In some cases this can be caused by wearing your hair in a pony tail, in your case it's caused by the weight of the extensions. Over a long period of time, this pulling stress can cause the follicle to atrophy and stop producing normal hairs. Depending on the intensity and duration of the stress the follicle may or may not recover. (You should consult a dermatologist to confirm this is really your problem.)

Follicle recovery
Hopefully you had the extensions removed in time and your follicles will recover and begin producing thick, strong hairs again. But if your follicles were permanently damaged, there's not much you can do. Sadly, there is no secret millionaire's product that can solve your problem; there is no known medical treatment for late-stage Traction Alopecia.

One thing MIGHT help increase hair strength, though is treatment with pure coconut oil. As the Brains have said before, that's one of the few natural oils that has been shown to penetrate the cortex and provide some strengthening effect to hair. It won't make your hair grow any thicker, but it might help protect your thinner weaker strands.

We wish you the best of luck write back and let us know how your hair turns out.

What Everyone Should Know About Straightening Irons

Kara's Question:
Hi, I'm in the market for a high-end straightening iron, and I feel completely overwhelmed by all the product choices out there! The major differences I see for most irons are the types of plates used, which include tourmaline/ceramic mix, ceramic, and metal plates. While I'm presuming it's the high heat (some heat up to 450F) that helps straighten the hair shaft, how do these different plates benefit the hair? Are these newer kinds of straighteners with the tourmaline and ceramic healthier for your hair? I'm looking for an iron that works well, but doesn't completely wreck and fry my hair shaft.

The Left Brain's Answer:
I agree, the number of choices for hair appliances is paralyzing! If it's any consolation, you don't have to pay too much attention to all the hype about the different types of ironing plates. While it's true that more expensive irons can be made from higher quality materials, that really just means that the heating element is more rugged and the plates are built to take wear and tear. Cheaper flat irons may have inferior plates that can't handle the heat and may snag your hair.

But whether it's tourmaline or ceramic, there's nothing about the composition of the plate material that makes it intrinsically healthier for your hair. And don't believe ANY of that crap about ionic straighteners. That's pure marketing hype without a shred of scientific validation.

The Beauty Brains bottom line
You'll need to pay a bit more for high quality construction but you don't need to pay extra for bogus scientific claims.

How To Kill Lice and Not Your Hair

Sandra Scratches Her Head:
I'm having a lice problem, I just wanted to know what's the most effective way to kill lice and nits and not dry or damage my hair in the process?? Thanx!!

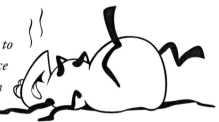

The Left Brain's Louse-y Reply:
Sorry to hear about your lice infestation problem, Sandra. Unfortunately, it's a pretty common problem. There are many other parasites that I'd prefer to have! But before I talk about a cure, here's a bit of background for those of you who may not be familiar with this problem:

Head lice are tiny crawling insects about the size of a sesame seed or smaller. They have six clawed legs that they use to crawl over your hair; they cannot hop, jump, or fly. Lice lay eggs, also known as Nits, which they glue to individual hair shafts. Lice live only on humans, not pets, and (here's the best part) they FEED ON HUMAN BLOOD!

Nit picking
The good news is that there several Over-The-Counter drug products that are effective against lice and nits. The bad news is, these products contain isopropyl alcohol which can dry your hair. There are "natural" lice cures but there is little or no data to prove these are effective. The safest and most sure way to get rid of lice and not damage your hair is to use a lice comb, but this is a very extremely tedious process.

Recently, there was a study done by researchers at the University of Utah in which they created a steam cleaning device (a cross between a vacuum cleaner and a hair dryer) to kill lice. This could prove pretty interesting.

Which treatment method is best for you? Rather than recount all the pros and cons of each method here, we'll point you to Head Lice.org for a very through question and answer page that you should find helpful. And if you do decide to use the lice-killing shampoo please make sure you follow that with a good conditioner to counteract the drying effects of the alcohol. Good luck!

The Cause Of Smelly Hair Syndrome

Betty's got a problem:
Hello! I am so GLAD I found you! I have had this problem now for about 3 months. I wash and condition my hair on a daily basis and by the middle of the day my hair has a sweaty, muggy smell. I just can't describe it, it just smells! Even worse when I'm running late in the morning and I am not able to wash my hair I could smell that sweaty, muggy smell throughout the day. I there anything I can do to stop this?

The Left Brain responds:
Betty, I had never heard of this problem before so I was surprised when I found out that you're not the only one who suffers from hair malodor. A quick search turned up several discussion boards on smelly hair. There's even a website that specializes in Smelly Hair.

What Causes Smelly Hair?
They claim the problem is a fungus that grows on oily scalps. That sounds plausible since the odor you describe as sweaty and muggy could be caused by microbial growth. I know that sometimes the towel I used to dry my hair develops a funky smell kind of like the one you describe. That happens when it doesn't dry out completely, so I assume there's some mildew or similar organism that responsible. If I don't notice it right way, that mildew odor transfers from the towel to my hair. Could this be the cause of your problem too?

What can you do about it?

Smellyscalp.com says use an antimicrobial shampoo. That certainly could help. You can also try changing your towel and your pillow case. If that doesn't work, you might try shaving your head, like Britney. (Just kidding!) You could also try using a product like the Stila hair refresher, but that will just cover up the odor. It won't address the source of the problem.

We hope this helps, and if you want more, try some of these the top 10 tips for stopping smelly hair on the next page.

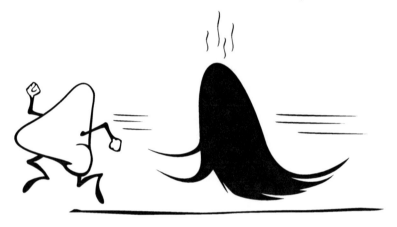

10 Tips to Stop Smelly Hair

Our good friend at the excellent "Are You A Beauty" blog has a great post about neutralizing hair odors. She gives a couple of great product suggestions, but we thought we'd look at all the ways you can use to stop smelly hair.

1. Wash and condition your hair
Yes it's a lot of work but that's really the most thorough way to get your hair clean.

2. Use hair wipes
Like Are You A Beauty suggests, you can use wipes made especially for hair like Ted Gibson's.

3. Use a hair fragrance
Beauty likes the one from Cleanperfume.com. If you don't mind spending $39.00. Ouch!

4. Spritz your hair with your own perfume
If you can't find a "real" hair fragrance just improvise with your fave perfume. Don't use too much!

5. Use a powder shampoo
Pssst anyone? Or maybe Batiste? Just spray 'em in and brush 'em out.

6. Use a leave-in conditioner or combing cream
A touch of conditioner can mask icky odors.

7. Do a speedy, secret sink wash
Wet your hands, take a TINY dab of liquid soap, and run your fingers through your hair. Caution: this doesn't work on all hairstyles.

8. Wipe your hair with a dryer sheet
It's better than smelling like smoke AND you'll get rid of embarrassing static cling.

9. Try a little Febreze on your brush
At least we THINK this might work. Better check with the manufacturer before you try this one at home!

10. Use an antimicrobial shampoo
This can help if you have Smelly Scalp Syndrome which is caused by scalp fungus or bacteria. Yuck!

Chapter 3
Hair Myths

How To Tell If You're Spending Too Much On Conditioner

Kathy's question:
I would like to know if spending more money on conditioners is worth it for increasing the strength of your hair. As a science teacher I would like to be able to explain why conditioners increase the strength of hair, and why the more expensive ones should work better!

The Right Brain's headstrong reply:
Kathy, from one science professional to another, we can tell you that expensive does NOT always mean better when it comes to hair and skin care products But to explain further, we'll have to fill you in on how conditioners work.

How do conditioners strengthen hair?

The outer layer of the hair consists of overlapping scales called cuticles. These cuticle are like the shingles on the roof of your house – they protect what's beneath it. As your hair is damaged from washing and drying and combing and brushing and perming and coloring, the cuticle starts to wear away. When this happens your hair is broken more easily.

Conditioners strengthen hair two ways. The most important thing they do is to smooth the cuticle and help keep it in place. The "strengthening" effect can be shown by measuring combing force. The other effect is internal. Some material, like panthenol, penetrate into the cortex, the middle part of the hair. By interacting with the proteins in the cortex, these conditioners can improve the tensile strength of hair. This type of strength is measured with an instrument that pulls on individual hair fibers (after they've been removed from your head, of course!) and measures how much force it takes for the hairto break. If you want to learn more, you can read our post on measuring hair breakage.

Are expensive conditioners better?

So do expensive conditioners strengthen hair better than cheap ones? Not necessarily. The very, very cheap conditioners typically rely on one or two conditioning agents to do the job. And they usually can't afford to use silicones, which are among the most effective smoothing agents. So, chances are, if you're only spending a buck or two on your conditioner, you're not getting the best product.

But once you get up to the $4 or $5 conditioners, the differences in strengthening are less significant. For example, Pantene and Tresemme are among the best conditioners we've ever tested and they're certainly not that expensive. Most mid or high priced conditioners will do a pretty good job of lubricating your hair to prevent breakage.

Can a conditioner be TOO expensive?

What about the conditioners that are $30 per bottle? They use the same basic types of ingredients as products that are $10 or less. They may cost 3 times more but they certainly don't strengthen your hair 3 times more! But as we always say, you should buy what you like and what you can afford. If you really like the way Frederic Fekkai's Overnight Hair Repair makes your hair feel, and you can afford the $195 per bottle then go for it. (Yes that's right – it's a $200 conditioner!) But don't buy it just because you think that it will make your hair stronger than another less expensive brand.   It won't.

The Beauty Brains bottom line

Picking the right conditioner is a very personal thing. There are literally thousands of combinations of ingredients out there and it's tough to know which one is best for you. So talk to your friends who have similar hair types. Or just experiment until you find something that feels good. But DON'T be tricked into spending more money than you want to.

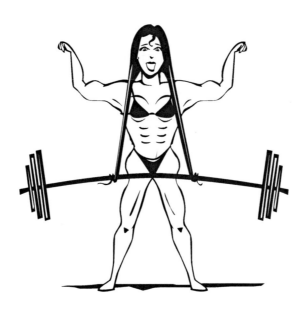

Will Copper Stop Your Dandruff?

Meg's brushing up on dandruff:
*I just bought copper-infused hair brush that supposedly gets rid of dandruff.
Will it really work?*

The Left Brain's flaky reply:
Meg is talking about the Goody "Styling Therapy - Reduce Dandruff
- Copper Infused" hairbrush. It claims to be "Infused with copper-plated
bristles, this brush kills 88% of the fungus that causes dandruff and dry, flaky
scalp; destroys bacteria and fungus associated with common scalp conditions.
Copper is proven to kill the leading cause of dandruff."

I can't find any credible research to show that a brush made with copper can
fight dandruff. But there is a kernel of truth behind their claims. It is well
known that metal salts of pyrithione are effective dandruff control agents.
Zinc Pyrithione, for example, is widely used in commercial dandruff
shampoos. There have been studies (see Nature and Pubmed) that show
copper salts may have some effect, but zinc salts are by far the most effective.
If a copper version worked better, trust me, big companies like P&G would
find a way to sell that in a product.

Even if copper ions are effective, it's highly unlikely that a copper brush
could provide enough scalp contact to deliver any sort of anti-fungal effect.
I say you're much better off using products like Head and Shoulders, Selsin
Blue, or Nizoral.

Why Do Gray Hairs Look And Feel Different

Trisha's question:
In a previous post you mentioned that gray hair looks gray because it has lost its melanin, which gives hair its pigment. What`s the biology involved with that? What actually causes hair to lose its melanin? And is there anything we can do to slow the process down? And why do my gray hairs seem more kinky and unruly compared to the rest of my hair?

The Left Brain's Response:
Melanin is a pigment that is naturally produced in the hair follicle and "injected" into the hair fibers as the protein is formed and pushed out of the head. It's the same kind of melanin that gives your skin its color. There are two basic types of melanin (eumelanin and pheomelanin) that are responsible for every hair color from brown and black to blond and red.

No one knows why hair follicles stop producing melanin. Genetics mostly. There just gets to be a point where the melanocytes (the melanin producing cells) just stop producing. Thus you get gray hair.

Slowing the process? No one has figured this one out just yet. And the truth is that only the pharmaceutical companies would be looking for the solution anyway. Cosmetic companies focus on things that do not react with your body. I'm not sure if there will be a solution to this problem anytime soon. (By the way, there are products out there like Reminex that claim to restore melanin production but we've seen no data to indicate they really work.)

There is no solid data to show that gray hair has a different physical structure that makes it feel more kinky and unruly. In fact, we've seen experiments that show if you have people close their eyes they can not feel a difference between gray hair and "normal" hair. Why do people think gray hair is so different? There are probably two reasons: First, we know that as you age, the follicles produce less of their natural lubricating oils. That can make hair feel dry and coarse. Second, gray hairs are just easier to notice because of the color difference. Think about all the hairs on your head that are unruly but they are the same color as the rest of your hair so you don't notice them.

Are Silicones Bad For Your Hair?

Diane's Undaunted By Silicones For Silkier Hair:

The question of silicone's usefulness has long being a subject of intense debate, speculation and confusion in Long Hair Community. As a consequence, a lot of members in Long Hair Community are wary of using silicone-heavy products, such as Pantene conditioner. Dimethicone, Cyclomethicone and whatnot are allegedly harder to rinse out, therefore build-up occurs faster than a silicone-free hair regimen.

As for me, I love how cones smooth and soften my hair big time - while in shower. Sadly, the miraculous silkiness vanishes as soon as my hair dries. So I use unrefined coconut oil to successfully add shine, softness and protection for my hair. My questions are these: Are 'cones really harder to rinse out? How do they work on hair? Do they dry hair out? And why does that wonderful silkiness disappear when my hair dries? How do carrier oils like coconut oil, sweet almond oil compare to silicones?

The Right Brain Comments on 'Cones for Conditioning:

Diane, you raise some very good questions. In general, silicones work by covering hair with a thin hydrophobic (water-proof) coating. This coating serves several purposes, it helps reduce the porosity of the hair which makes it less likely to absorb humidity; it helps reduce moisture loss from the inside of the hair; and it lubricates the surface of the hair so it feel smoother and combs easier.

Properties of silicones

The properties vary depending on which particular silicone is in the formula. Some silicones do leave a heavy coating on the hair that can be hard to wash off. Others are very water soluble and don't buildup at all. Dimethicone, (sometimes called simethicone) for example, is the heaviest of all silicones used for hair care. It provides the most smoothing effect but it is also the hardest to wash out. Cyclomethicone on the other hand, gives great slippery feeling while you're rinsing your hair, but it quickly evaporates leaving nothing behind. This is probably what you're experiencing.

What about carrier oils, as you describe them? Some oils are effective conditioners. Take coconut oil, for example. While it doesn't provide the same surface smoothing as silicones, it has been shown to penetrate hair and plasticize the cortex, making hair stronger. (This isn't true of all natural oils however.) So oils are useful ingredients but they're not direct replacements for silicones.

The Beauty Brains bottom line
It's tough to tell simply from reading the label because there are so many types of silicones and they can be used in combination with each other. You can't simply say all silicones are bad. Some women will find silicones too heavy for their hair, others will love the soft, conditioned feel they provide. You'll have to experiment to find what's right for you. Good luck!

Can You Really Rebuild Your Hair?

The Glitterati asks:
What is the deal with "restructuring" treatments for hair? I mean, I get that the vague concept is to "restore proteins" to your hair or some gobbledy-gook, but isn't hair essentially dead? Can a restructuring treatment really force-feed amino acids or whatever into our manes?

And The Left Brain responds:
By the tone of your question, a certain level of skepticism on your part is evident. We here at the Beauty Brains love that! And it's a good thing because the idea of being able to slather on a hair restructuring treatment to actually re-form hair is ridiculous. True, hair is made of amino acids and putting them on hair may provide some minor benefit. But it won't restructure, restore or rebuild the hair. This would be a bit like trying to repair a weather-

worn Kate Spade bag by pouring a basket of thread and fabric on it. Sure, the stylish sack is made of thread and fabric but you can't just randomly put them on and expect to get a new purse.

Restructured hair?

It's the same way with hair and amino acids. To really restructure the hair, the amino acids would have to be chemically arranged in a specific way. This arrangement can only be done in the hair follicle when the hair is growing. After that, nothing can be done except coat the hair with a good conditioner that mitigates some of the signs of damage. So, what are these restructuring treatments? In essence, they are just glorified rinse-out conditioners. Just take a look at the ingredients. Here is Tricomin Restructuring Conditioner:

Purified Water, Glyceryl Stearate, PEG-100 Stearate, Stearamidopropyl Dimethylamine, Cetyl Alcohol, Propylene Glycol, Stearyl Alcohol, Dimethicone, Triamino Copper Nutritional Complex (see product information for ingredients), Hydroxyethylcellulose, Panthenol, Aloe Vera Gel, Soydimonium Hydroxypropyl Hydrolyzed Wheat Protein, Hydrolyzed Keratin, Citric Acid, Methylparaben, Fragrance, Disodium EDTA, Propylparaben, Peppermint Oil, Tocopheryl Acetate, Cholecalciferol, Retinyl Palmitate, Vegetable Oil, FD&C Blue 1, D&C Red 33

The rules of cosmetic labeling require that ingredients are listed in order of concentration above 1%. In general, the more of an ingredient in the formula, the more impact it has on the product. The ingredients near the end of the list are just put in there to make a nice marketing story or are color, fragrance or preservatives.

In the Tricomin formula, some of the main working ingredients are *Stearamidopropyl Dimethylamine, Cetyl Alcohol, Stearyl Alcohol, and Dimethicone.* But then take a look at a regular rinse-out conditioner. Say Pantene Pro-V Conditioner, Smooth and Sleek

Water, Stearyl Alcohol, Cyclopentasiloxane, Cetyl Alcohol, Stearamidopropyl Dimethylamine, Glutamic Acid, Dimethicone, Benzyl Alcohol, Fragrance, Panthenyl Ethyl Ether, EDTA, Panthenol, Methylchloroisothiazolinone, Methylisothiazolinone

Notice any similarities?? The main working ingredients here are *Stearyl Alcohol, Cyclopentasiloxane, Cetyl Alcohol, Stearamidopropyl Dimethylamine, and Dimethicone.*

The Beauty Brains bottom line
Both of these are good conditioners. But the Restructuring Conditioner will not rebuild your hair any better than a standard rinse-out formula. And it certainly won't rebuild your hair better than thread and fabric would rebuild a worn out Kate Spade.

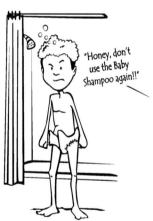

"Honey, don't use the Baby Shampoo again!!"

Is Sulfate-Free Baby Shampoo Good For Adult Hair?

Shiraune Says:
In viewing your site I have become an instant fan. I appreciate the unbiased information you provide here. My question is are baby shampoos sufficient enough to clean adult hair? I know they are SLS free and have been looking for this type of shampoo to minimize the drying effect from SLS poos.

The Left Brain Responds:
Thanks for the kind words about the blog. We always try to provide helpful, unbiased information when answering your questions. And your question in particular is a good one because there is a lot of misinformation out there about Sodium Lauryl Sulfate (SLS) and shampoo.

Is SLS bad?

First of all, don't believe all the urban legends about SLS causing cancer or being bad for you because it's used in garage cleaners. We've blogged about SLS and pointed out that these myths have been debunked. Most people can use Sodium Lauryl Sulfate or Ammonium Lauryl Sulfate shampoos without any problem whatsoever.

BUT, some people do find that SLS can dry out their scalp. Those people should consider SLS's milder cousin SLES (short for Sodium Lauryl Ether Sulfate) or they should consider using sulfate-free shampoos.

Are baby shampoos good cleansers?

Baby shampoos are good examples of sulfate-free formulas. Instead of SLS they contain materials known as amphoteric surfactants that are less drying to skin and milder to the eye. (Hence the "no more tears" claim of many baby shampoos.)

The downside to these types of formulations is that they don't clean as well as the stronger detergent systems. While SLS is a VERY good cleansing agent that can remove sweat, dirt, styling product residue and scalp oils, baby shampoo formulas are not so effective.

Why not baby yourself?

Is this a problem? It depends. If you're using a ton of styling product you might have to shampoo your hair multiple times with baby shampoo to get it as clean as an SLS-based product. That's not such a bad trade off if your scalp is really dried out. I recommend trying baby shampoo for a week or two to see if you like the effect. If not, you can always switch back.

And if you've got money to burn, you can also check out the adult version of baby shampoos EN Joy Hydrating Shampoo, Back To Basics Color Protecting Shampoo, or even Paves.

Want to learn more? You can visit the Beauty Brains and read more of our blog posts about Sulfates.

For Seriously Tangled Hair - Don't Rely On Homemade Moisturizers

Jim's Got A Problem:

Here's my problem. I'm an "older" male who has kept his long hair. Now that I'm left with only about 26,000 hairs!! it's still long, curly … and once I spend 20 minutes in the shower with a ton of conditioner, looks great.

My hair is SO tangly that virtually every hair I have tangles with every other hair. After gobs of conditioner and 20 minutes in the shower separating every hair from every other hair - 2 days later it's a tangled mess again. I stopped using any shampoo or soap or anything (except conditioner) a long time ago. I've never coloured my hair or used any chemicals on it.

So - what's the most powerful, de-tangler you know of? I'd be prepared to use some spray on Teflon cookware product it that meant not having to slowly, slowly (from the bottom up naturally) separate every hair with tons of conditioner! Please help this super tangled guy!

The Right Brain Responds:

Jim, as always it's a pleasure to hear from our male readers. We just wish there was more we could do to help you.

What Makes Hair So Tangly?

It's possible that you have a medical condition that can cause hair to become excessively tangled. It's called Uncombable Hair Syndrome and it occurs when your hair shaft is more triangular than cylindrical. Without examining your hair, it's difficult to determine what your condition really is.

Would A Homemade Moisturizer Help?

Probably not, homemade products just aren't that powerful. There are plenty of good conditioners that should be sufficient to detangle "normal" hair. Fructis is a great product because it combines fatty alcohols and silicones in a very slippery formula. If you haven't tried that product, you might give it a shot. You might also try using a wide tooth pick in the shower to work the conditioner through your wet hair. Finally, you might also consider using a leave in conditioner in your hair at night to reducing tangling while you toss and turn in your sleep.

You've probably heard some of this advice in the long hair forums, but we hope some of this info helps.

Do You Really Need To Put Protein On Your Hair?

Doppleganger says:
I've been told that hair needs protein and moisturization to stay healthy. So, for protein I use Mane 'n Tail and for moisturization I use hair cholesterol products (like Le Kair, Queen Helene) and coconut oil. Is this good for my hair or can I be causing any kind of long term damage?

The Left Brain Replies:
Relax, Dop. These conditioners won't damage your hair. You might find that your hair is weighed down if you're using them all at once, but other than that they won't do anything bad to your hair. So if you like the way these conditioners make your hair feel, then keep using them anyway you like. The real question here is, does hair really need protein and moisturization? The answer is yes and no.

YES, hair needs moisturization
That just means you need to keep your hair from drying out. That's the whole idea behind conditioners. You can moisturize by adding water (which doesn't

really stay in your hair very long) or you can moisturize by fighting the effects of dryness. That's what any good conditioner does. Conditioners, like Le Kair and Queen Helene, work by smoothing the outer layers of your hair, the part called the cuticle. Cuticles are like shingles on top of a roof. If you don't keep them "glued down" they tend to come loose and fall off. When ever you're doing anything to your hair (including washing, drying, styling, or coloring), your causing some degree of damage to those cuticles. What a good conditioner does is smooth the cuticles, forming a protective layer over them so they don't become as damaged.

NO, hair doesn't need protein

Although, hair is made of protein, it's dead. So putting protein on top f the protein in your hair doesn't really make it "healthy." But the right kind of proteins used at the right levels can act as a conditioning agent that can form a protective film on the hair. So it's not that your hair needs protein, it's that it needs SOMETHING to form that protective layer. Proteins will do it to some extent, but there are other ingredients like fatty quaternium compounds or silicones, that will work even better. So protein conditioners like Mane 'n Tail are good for your hair, but not necessarily BECAUSE they contain protein. We've written other posts about protein if you'd like to read more.

The Beauty Brains Bottom line

There are many, many great hair conditioners on the market that will moisturize your hair. Mane n' Tail, Le Kair, and Queen Helene won't do anything bad to you. The important thing is to find the ones that feel right for your hair and that you can afford. But don't worry too much about special ingredients like proteins. Oh, and by the way, the coconut oil you're using has an added benefit. It penetrates through the cuticle to strengthen the inside side part of the hair called the cortex. But that's a topic for another post.

Cosmetic Safety - Will Hair Dye Give You Cancer?

Every so often you hear about how chemicals in your cosmetics are responsible for cancer, birth defects or even autism. Unfortunately, the sources for these conclusions are rarely cited and when they are, they are typically a biased political committee or marketing group.

This article about hair dye and cancer caught my eye. Reading the title is downright scary "Can dyeing your hair really give you cancer?" The article continues to discuss a major conference that is being held in Belfast in which they'll discuss the long-term link between bladder cancer and people with dyed hair. It even states

> *Evidence exists to indicate regular and long term use of hair*
> *dyes can be associated with the development of the cancer which*
> *kills more than 4,000 in the UK each year.*

Now, if this article was all you read on the subject, you might conclude that hair dye causes bladder cancer. You might also get the impression that experts are in agreement. After all, they did get their information from Questor a European Environmental Research Centre.

Being the skeptical Beauty Brain that I am, I went to see what the medical journals had to say on the subject. A search of 'hair dye' resulted in 649 hits. The most current research is most useful and for answering questions like these, review articles are best. Review articles are designed to summarize all the work that has been published before.

Does hair dye cause cancer?
This article about hair dye and cancer published in late 2006 in the Journal of Toxicology and Environmental Health concludes

> *Results for bladder cancer studies suggest that subsets of the*
> *population may be genetically susceptible to hair dye exposures, but*

these findings are based on small subgroups in one well-designed case-control study. Replication of these findings is needed to determine whether the reported associations are real or spurious.

This is a bit different than the definitive bladder cancer/hair dye link suggested in the newspaper article. Essentially the researchers say certain genetically predisposed people may have issues, but even this isn't a certainty. A more thorough study is needed. But the important implication is that for most people, this isn't a problem. Hair dye will not cause cancer.

The Beauty Brains bottom line
What you read, see or hear in the mainstream media rarely tells the whole story. When it comes to issues about health and safety you would not be wrong to immediately reject their conclusions. If you want to know the real story do a little research from yourself using the least biased sources you can find. Research in this case would find that the majority of research shows no established link between hair dye and cancer. So, feel free to color with abandon. I know I will.

For a more thorough summary of the cancer/hair color research look at this article published in The Journal of the American Medical Association*.

*http://jama.ama-assn.org/cgi/content/abstract/293/20/2516

Chapter 4
Skin Treatment - From Silly to Sublime

The Best Skin Moisturizing Oils In The World

Pamela Ponders:

Since the weather is getting drier, I've decided to look for some cuticle treaments to help them from drying. I've noticed that a lot of them include very similar ingredients, like jojoba oil, apricot kernel oil, shea butter, and in particular sweet almond oil and lavender oil. Do these ingredients really help to moisturize and what exactly do they do? I've noticed a lot of body care products emphasize shea butter. I've also noticed them some body lotions have coconut oil in it, is this another beneficial ingredient?

The Right Brain Responds:

All the oils you mentioned can moisturize skin - but they're not the BEST moisturizers. What are the best, you ask? Ah, that is the question. But first you have to sit through this quick explanation:

How oils moisturize

Moisture evaporates from your skin by slipping though tiny cracks and fissures oils form a barrier layer on top of the skin that prevents the water molecules from escaping. It's all about stopping evaporation! This property is called occlusivity and it's measured by a rating called Transepidermal Water Loss, or TEWL. (pronounced "tool.") The TEWL value has been measured for various oils, and the ones that have the highest rating (in other words, the ones that stop the most water from escaping your skin) are as follows:

Top 5 moisturizing oils
1. **Petroleum Jelly** (in a minimum concentration of 5%, reduces TEWL by more than 98%)
2. **Lanolin**
3. **Mineral oil**
4. **Dimethicone** (a type of silicone)
5. **Others including other oils** (like coconut), fatty alcohols, and waxes

The Beauty Brains bottom line

Some of the other oils you mentioned are still beneficial - they can make skin feel softer and smoother. But if you really want to keep your skin moist, you need to reduce evaporation with one of these top 5.

3 Reasons Why Hand and Face Moisturizers Should Be Different

Kay's Question:
Is there a difference between moisturizers for your hands and for your face? Relatedly, is there a reason to use specially formulated anti-wrinkle creams rather than ordinary moisturizers that you would use on your hands?

The Right Brain saves face:
Yes, Kay, this is one of these cases where there is some really science behind the marketing hype. Here's why facial lotions should be different than hand lotions:

1. Skin on hands and face are different
Skin is very thin on your face and thicker on your hands. Also, your hands don't (usually) develop acne or blackheads. Therefore, they need to be treated differently.

2. Drying conditions are different for hands and face
You may wash your hands in harsh soap many times a day; you may only wash your face once or twice with a gentle cleanser. Hands are in and out of dish water or laundry water, your face is not. The cumulative effect is that your hands can be much dryer, even cracked and bleeding, and therefore they need stronger moisturization.

3. Hands and face have different cosmetic needs
You might want to tighten the little crows feet wrinkles around your eyes but this isn't the case on your hands.

The Beauty Brains bottom line
For the reasons above and more, you need to use products designed to suit your skin's different needs. Hand lotions should be heavier barrier creams to protect from harsh conditions. Facial moisturizers should be lightweight, noncomedogenic, and may have film forming agents that tighten skin to

help reduce the appearance of fine lines and wrinkles. While hand and face products may share some of the same basic ingredients, the functions they need to perform can be significantly different. Using the right product on the right skin will give you better results.

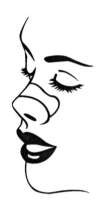

Do Pore Strips Really Work?

Anonymous Asks:
What can you tell us about Biore-type pore strips? It's strangely fascinating seeing all the crap come off on the strips, but is just a quick-fix that will actually make things worse in the long run?

The Right Brain Boasts About Biore:
A pore strip, like Biore's, is a very dramatic way to clean your pores. It works by adhering tightly to your skin so tightly that when you pull it off it also pulls out the oily, dirty gunk that is clogging your pores.

Pore strips really work
The cool thing is that you can actually SEE the pore poop stuck to the strip after you take it off. The first time the Beauty Brains tried this product they sat staring transfixed at the forest of tiny nasal pore discharges dotting the landscape of the freshly spent pore strip. Some white heads were barely visible to the naked eye; other black heads where ominously thick and dark. We still get shivers just thinking about it.

Even if you don't feel you need them, we recommend trying pore strips as an experiment just so you can see for yourself.

The problem with pore strips
When used correctly, Pore Strips can be a powerful weapon in your battle against blackheads. But don't use them too often because they can irritate

your skin. Three times per week max, that's the limit. Any more than that and you risk damaging your skin. You should heed the warnings on the box about not using them on any area other than the nose and not to use them over inflamed, swollen, sunburned, or excessively dry skin. If you use pore strips too often, they can actually irritate your skin and trigger more breakouts.

5 Things You Need To Know About Retin-A

Beauty Bug begs an answer:
I'm currently reading Free Gift with Purchase, by Jean Godfrey-June, the beauty editor for Lucky. The books says that Retin-A helps with wrinkles and Beauty Bug wants the Beauty Brains to comment. Does Retin-A really get rid of wrinkles?

The Left Brain responds:
What is Retin-A
Retin-A is the brand name of a prescription drug called Tretinoin which is a derivative of vitamin A. In 1971, the FDA approved the topical application of Tretinoin to treat acne and sun damaged skin. This drug works by irritating the skin, which triggers the basal layer to produce fresh skin cells, thus increasing cell turnover. (Mmmm, turnover!) As new cells more rapidly replace the old ones, the skin takes on a younger, smoother appearance. So it does work, but there are a few issues you should be aware of.

5 Things You Need to Know About Retin-A
1. It's a prescription drug so you can only get it from your doctor.
2. It doesn't work over night. Wrinkles start to decrease or disappear after three to six months.
3. Some of the drug is absorbed into the body and may cause problems with pregnancy.
4. It can be so irritating that it burns and causes redness.
5. While it does help reduce wrinkles that doesn't mean it gets rid of ALL your wrinkles. As they say, results will vary.

The Beauty Brains bottom line

Unlike so many wrinkle creams, this drug has been proven to really do something (despite the issues cited above.) And don't fall for the claims of other products that are really just regular cosmetics with Vitamin A derivatives.

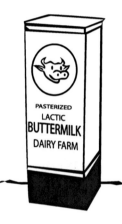

An Inexpensive, Natural Wrinkle Remover, From The Dairy Case

Michelle's got milk: *I am 54 years young and when I was 22 I was told to put buttermilk on my face to get rid of wrinkles. I've been using it ever since and there is no question that my skin looks much younger than women my age. I have also stayed out of the sun and don't smoke and today I also use pricey beauty products like ReVive and Origins. Do you think it's buttermilk that's keeping my skin wrinkle free?*

The Right Brain goes sour:

Michelle, thanks so much for your email. We had to edit it to fit today's post, but we've started a forum thread with your entire email in case anyone's interested in learning more. Now on to your answer...

Could buttermilk be responsible for your youthful appearance?

Mmmmmmaybe. But doubtful. Here's why.

What the heck is buttermilk, anyway?

For those of you who aren't up to speed on your dairy products, buttermilk is a thickened, sour type of milk that is made by adding bacteria to regular milk. The bacteria cause fermentation which changes the milk sugar (aka lactose) into lactic acid. Sound familiar? It should! Lactic acid is an alpha-hydroxyacid (or AHA) the same chemical that's used in anti-aging lotions to exfoliate your skin. Unfortunately, it doesn't look like buttermilk is better than lotions you can buy.

Why isn't buttermilk better?

Milk   contains 4 to 6% lactose. When it's converted to buttermilk, you end up with about 3 or 4% lactic acid. Lactic acid skin creams contain about 12% lactic acid, about 3 times as much as buttermilk. So while it's theoretically possible that buttermilk could be helping, you'd probably see more benefit from a relatively inexpensive lactic acid cream like Lac-hydrin.

So, if it's not the buttermik, why does your skin look good?

There could be several other reasons you skin looks so good. First, genetics plays a large role in the health of your skin. It might also be your healthy lifestyle. By staying out of the sun and not smoking you've avoided two of the major causes of premature aging. Finally, you said that you're using other beauty products like Revive and Origins along with the buttermilk. If any of these products contain sunscreen that could be prevent your skin from aging too. But the important thing is - keep up whatever you're doing. It's working for you!

And if anyone is still interested in buttermilk but you don't like the stench of sourmilk on your face (and gee, who doesn't want that??) you also might try Burt's Bees Buttermilk Lotion. It's 98.31% natural so it MUST be good. Right?

Are Oral Supplements Good For My Skin?

Cheong Asks:
Do oral skin supplements like Imedeen really work?? I do believe that you are what you eat, and a healthy diet does help your skin, but can taking things like collagen or bird's nest soup or ginseng really give you better skin??

The Left Brain Begets:
Thanks for a great question. We get these kind all the time asking if various food supplements are going to help skin, hair, weight loss, and even longevity.

Supplements are unregulated...that's bad
The claims on some of these things are so wild, it seems that just popping a pill everyday should fix every problem you've got. Of course, this is nonsense. Remember, food and health supplements are NOT REGULATED. They can say ANYTHING they want, even if it is a LIE, and no one will likely do anything about it. So, when it comes to supplements the first reaction for every Beauty Brainiac should be one of skepticism.

What's Imedeen's story?
So, what about Imedeen? Imedeen is basically a skincare supplement that includes proteins, polysaccharides, vitamin C and other "free radical scavengers". According to the company...

> *Imedeen Time Perfection is state-of-the-art skincare based on natural ingredients that are scientifically documented to visibly reduce signs of ageing from within and to help defend against new signs of ageing from forming.*

And after just 2 to 3 months of use, you are supposed to SEE results. Hope in a bottle is finally here! Yeah, right. Although, in the event that you don't notice anything after a month of use, they include this disclaimer...

As with any nutritional supplement, the response will vary from person to person, and depends on skin condition, general health, diet, environment and other factors.

Which basically means if it doesn't work for you, then there must be something wrong with YOU.

First, the notion that what you eat affects the condition of your skin may make sense but few, if any studies have shown any link between diet and skin conditions. Unless you are malnourished, there will not be any noticeable difference in your skin. It's highly unlikely that using this supplement will have any noticeable effect.

Imedeen makes a lot of strong claims
Next, let's look at some of their specific claims for this supplement.
1. Instantly begins to neutralise the skin-degrading processes
2. Significantly improves the skin's moisture balance
3. Visibly reduces the appearance of fine lines and wrinkles
4. Diminishes visibility of dilated capillaries and age spots
5. Leaves the skin with a brighter, more youthful and even complexion
6. Helps shield and defend the vital structural elements of the skin against future degradation

But there's very little supportive data
What do these claims really mean? The first claim sounds compelling but it doesn't really mean that much. "Instantly begins?" Why doesn't it "Instantly neutralise"? And notice how they don't spell out what the "skin-degrading processes" are? What could they possibly mean? They are hoping you'll make up something that you believe is "skin-degrading" and believe that this stuff stops it.

The second claim doesn't make much sense either. What is the "skin's moisture balance"? The only factors that can affect this are the condition of your skin and environmental factors like temperature and humidity.

What about the rest of the claims? Reduce fine lines and wrinkles? These claims come from their scientific data. But a study that they reference as proof clearly concludes that after 3 months there are "NO SIGNIFICANT EFFECTS detected." It is only after 9 MORE MONTHS of an uncontrolled study that the Imedeen shows any effect. Unfortunately, with an uncontrolled study there is no way to tell what caused the positive results they saw. This is extremely weak data!

The sixth and final claim also is pretty worthless. How do you prove that you "shield and defend" against future skin damage? You can't! What a bunch of marketing gobbly gook.

The most outrageous part of this supplement is how much it costs. According to our friends at beauty.com, a box of Imedeen contains 60 tablets (1 month of treatment) that cost $70. So , you'll have to buy $210 worth of supplements to see any effect, if there is any effect. In fact, since their own study says it'll take 9 months to see a benefit, that will set you back a whopping $630! Is that worth it to you?

The Beauty Brains bottom line

Imedeen has some slick marketing and even a couple of "studies" to back up what they say. But with the prices they charge, the weakness of their data and the fact that you'll still have to apply sunscreens and moisturizers, this doesn't seem like a smart purchase at all. You'd be better off saving up your money for plastic surgery. And as far as collagen, bird's nest soup or ginseng giving you better skin…I don't think so.

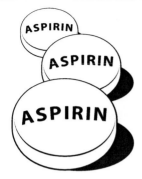

Is An Aspirin Mask Good For Skin?

Ivy Asks About Aspirin:

I've been preparing to write about Aspirin Masks. The mask is prepared by crushing four aspirins and mixing it with a bit of water to create a paste. Then it's smeared over one's face. Do you know anything about this do-it-yourself cosmetic?

The Right Brain Responds:

Aspirin masks seem to be all the rage these days, but we can't find any evidence that they're worth the effort. Here's why:

What is aspirin?

The active ingredient in aspirin is the drug called Acetylsalicylic Acid. After you swallow an aspirin tablet it travels to your small intestine where this ingredient is broken down to create to Salicylic Acid. Salicylic Acid, or Sal Acid as it's referred to, is the form of the drug that actually reduces pain, fever, etc.

Now, Sal Acid also belongs to the class of chemicals known as Beta Hydroxy Acids, or BHAs. BHAs are similar to AHAs (Alpha Hydroxy Acids). Both BHAs and AHAs are known for their ability to help slough off dead skin cells when applied topically. Are you beginning to see the connection between aspirin and facial masks?

Why aspirin isn't good for your skin

In theory, crushing aspirin tablets and rubbing them on your face COULD be beneficial because you're delivering a skin smoothing BHA, right? Well, not exactly.

You're really delivering Acetylsalicylic Acid to the skin - NOT Salicylic Acid, which is the active BHA. And just rubbing the Acetyl verision on your skin won't make it convert to the Sal Acid version. Ok, maybe SOME of the acid is present in the Sal version, but it certainly isn't an optimized dose.

The Beauty Brains bottom line
Putting crushed aspirin on your face might have SOME benefit, but if you really want a skin smoothing BHA treatment, just buy one of the many Sal Acid products on the market. In this case the home-made remedy doesn't appear as effective as the chemist-made one.

A Safe Way to Make Your Skin Look Brighter and Younger

Margaret and Betty are inquisitive about Definity:
Margaret says Definity works great for her but she wants to know if all the roducts in the line are basically the same; Betty is worried that Definity's not safe because she heard it contains hydroquinone.

The Right Brain provides this definitive response:
P&G must be doing a good job of marketing their Olay line because we get a lot of questions about Definity. So, we present a double dose of Definity: In Part 1 we explain how the products work; in Part 2, we'll talk about how the products in the line are different from one another.

What Does Definity Do?
According to P&G, Definity "fights what ages you most: discoloration, dullness, brown spots, and fights wrinkles." The fighting wrinkles stuff is pretty standard in beauty creams. If you're hydrating the skin (especially if you're using a film forming agent that helps hide fine lines) you can support anti-wrinkle claims. The interesting aspect of Definity is that it claims to make the skin more luminous because it gets rid of darkness and dullness.

How Does Definity Make Skin Luminous?
Skin lightening claims like these normally involve hydroquinone, a skin bleaching agent that's come under fire for safety reasons. Fortunately,

Definity doesn't contain hydroquinone. Instead, it uses N-acetyl glucosamine, chemical that inhibits glycosylation of pro-tyrosinase. (Relax, that just means it prevents the kind of chemical reactions that make liver spots and freckles.) N-acetyl glucosamine (or NAG as it's known) is not as effective as hydroquinone, but it's safer to use.

Sound too good to be true? Check out the multiple clinical test results that show glucosamine effectively prevents dark age spots. And if dark spots are reduced, skin will look lighter and more luminous.

Of course, the question is, how MUCH improvement will you really see. The only way to tell for sure is to try the product. But at least Olay has done their homework and formulated a product line that's based on science, not snake oil.

The Beauty Brains bottom line
Definity does contain an ingredient proven to lighten skin. Of course, that doesn't guarantee that you'll notice a difference yourself. It's a bit expensive at $22 for 1.7 ounces, but at least their claims are based on real science.

Is Definity Decidely Different? - Part 2

In Part 1 we explained how Olay's Definity is based on real science that, at least theoretically, can reduce dark age spots and make skin look more luminous.

In Part 2 we examine the different products in the Definity line. There are six altogether: Definity Foaming Moisturizer, Foaming moisturizer with UV absorber, Correcting Protective Lotion (or is that Protecting Corrective Lotion?); Intense Hydrating cream; Illuminating Cream Cleanser; and Pore Redefining Scrub.

Why six products? Is it because P&G is satanically trying to remind you of 666, the mark of the beast? Oh wait, that's a myth; we already proved that P&G isn't run by Satanists. So there must be another reason that they'd offer six different products. Actually we can think of three reasons and they all boil down to trying to catch the attention of you, the Shopper:

1. Providing solutions to multiple skin care problems
Four of the products are moisturizers; two of those contain a UV absorber. The other two products are cleaners. By offering different benefits across their product line, they appeal to women seeking solutions to different skin care problems.

2. Offering similar benefits in different formats
Maybe you like to put on a heavier moisturizer at night, so you use the Intensive Cream. I like to use a lighter product in the morning so I buy the Foaming Moisturizer. By offering similar products in different formats, they appeal to a broader audience.

3. Creating a stronger shelf presence
Let's face it, cosmetic companies are in business to sell products. To sell products they have to make them available to consumers, which means getting their products onto store shelves. And the more products on shelf, the easier it is for consumers to find them. This is a strategy known as "brand blocking." Companies put as many of their products together on shelf as possible to create a more impactful impression. So one of the reasons there are six different Definity products is that it makes good business sense.

Ok, to be fair to Olay, they don't say that you have to use all six products. They recommend using a cleanser, a moisturizer and a sunscreen moisturizer. But wait. That means you're using two moisturizers. One of which Protects and Corrects and the other Perfects and Deflects. Or is that Detects and Reflects? Connects and Rejects? Arrrrrh! This is confusing!

The Beauty Brains bottom line

Let's keep it simple: if you're curious, pick a Definity moisturizer and cleanser that you like and give them a try. If you don't notice a difference after a few weeks, don't buy them again. Whew!

Cure Warts With Duct Tape

Here's a great tip for the Do-It-Yourself crowd:
Duct tape can cure warts!

Yes, it's true, according to Anthony J. Mancini M.D., an associate professor at Northwestern University's School of Medicine Children's Memorial Hospital in Chicago. Dr. Mancini says he uses duct tape as an inexpensive and relatively painless way to treat warts. He has his patients apply the duct tape over the wart, leave it on for about a week, remove the tape, and then file the wart with an emory board. It's that easy.

How does it work?
But how can such a simple household item treat a sustained viral infection?

No one knows, at least not for sure. But theoretically the tape could be debriding, or stripping the dead skin from the wart and carrying the wart virus along with it. That's kind of how other wart therapies work. (Like the Compound W or Kryoderm freezing technique). Another possible mechanism is that occluding skin with duct tape somehow triggers the patient's immune system to fight the virus. There's no solid data to support this theory but doctors do use immunotherapy

Do Shave Minimizing Lotions Work?

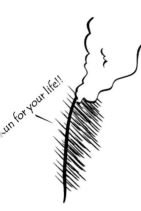

un for your life!!

Glitterati want to know:
Do "hair growth inhibiting" products like Jergen's Shave Minimizing Lotion really work?

**The Right Beauty Brain's
Rigorously Researched Response:**
Uh, not really.

The hairy truth

These products don't reduce the rate at which hair grows and they don't even do much to reduce the hair that's already grown out! We agree with the assessment of the folks over at Hairfacts, whom we quote:

> **Does it remove or reduce hair?** No.
> **Does it make hair appear less noticeable?** Maybe.
> **Does daily use make shaving easier?** Quite probably.
> **Does daily use allow you to shave less often?** Maybe.
> **Is it better at softening hair than any other extra-strength moisturizer?** Not been proven.

This lotion contains a lot of heavy emollients (softeners) and a mild amount of an alkaline solution used to dissolve hair.

That pretty much sums it up. Products like the Jergen's lotion actually claim to help make hair softer, finer, and less noticeable. That does NOT mean they slow down how fast the hair grows back, which is what they imply. (By the way, we doubt that there is sufficient alkali in the lotion to make a difference because products like this are designed to be left on skin and true depilatories must be rinsed off because prolonged skin contact will cause irritation.)

Finally, as Hairfacts points out, "The only quantitative claim they need to back up is their claim that it lets you shave 'half as often'. If you shave every day or so, you might be able to go every other day or so."

The Beauty Brains bottom line
Sorry, looks like you'll have to keep shaving.

What's The Right Way To Apply Sunscreen?

Kim's Query:
My question is about sunscreen: On the bottle, it says to apply 15-30 minutes before sun exposure so the product can absorb. Say I apply sunscreen to my hands, wait half an hour, then wash them. Will the skin on my hands still be protected from the sun? Or do I need to apply again, and wait another 30 minutes?

The Right Brain's Solar-Powered Reply:
Kim, your question reminds us of the recent comment from Marcy who's husband believes that the big sunscreen companies tell us we have to apply more sunscreen just to boost sales. You haven't been hanging with Marcy's husband have you? We didn't think so, but we just had to ask.

First of all, if you're washing off the sunscreen you've already put on, it doesn't matter if you wait the 30 minutes or not. You've got to leave it on or it won't work. But if you're just concerned about protecting your hands, we wouldn't worry too much. You can apply sunscreen to your hands and then just carefully wash the palms so they don't feel greasy. That way the backs of your hands will be protected and there's little chance that your palms will get enough sun to cause a problem. But if you're still worried about it, you could always wear gloves at the beach like the Left Brain does!

Still confused about how to apply sunscreen? We'll pass on these sunscreen application tips from the American Academy of Dermatologists

3 simple steps to safer sun protection

1. Put on plenty: An ounce or so (the article says a shot glass full, hence today's picture) should about do it for the average person.

2. Soak it up: For maximum protection, wait for it to soak in before (15 to 30 minutes) before frolicking in the sun.

3. Frequent reapplication: Reapply often, at least every two hours.

Why is this last item so important? First, because the UV absorbing molecules can wear out over time so your protection level drops off. Second, because sweating, swimming, and towel drying can remove sunscreen from your skin's surface. Do you really have to put more on after only 2 hours? Apparently yes. Studies have shown that people who wait 2 and a half hours instead of 2, have a 5 times greater chance of burning.

Yes, this means you might go through an entire bottle of sunscreen during a day at the beach. But that's still cheaper than a visit to your friendly neighborhood dermatologist to have a spot of melanoma removed!

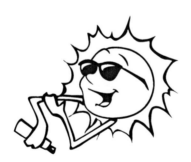

3 Ways To Tell If Your Sunscreen Is Bad

Catherine's Concerned About Sunscreen Efficacy: I've heard that when sunscreen/sunblock separates, it's no longer good. That shaking it up to remix it is basically wasted effort and applying it will do no good at all. Is this true? Can sunscreen go bad?

The Left Brain Concurs:
Sunscreen formulations are very sensitive creatures. Most UV absorbers are oil soluble, which means they have to be carefully emulsified to form stable mixtures with water. If the oil and water in the formula are not properly coupled together, the whole formula can go to hell pretty quickly. Here are 3 warning signs that your sunscreen has gone sour:

1. Weird consistency
The consistency of the product has changed over time and now it's too thick or too thin to spread properly. The spreadability of sunscreens is crucial to proper application and coverage. If it doesn't spread right, it won't work right.

2. Crystalization
The active ingredient has crystallized out, making the lotion feel gritty. When this happens the product is completely worthless. You can't fix that by shaking.

3. Separation
The product has separated into two different layers. Also not good. At worst, the active ingredient will partition into the oil phase and shaking it may or may not re-suspend it properly. At best, the water-resistance of the product may be compromised and it will wash off too easily. Either way, it's really not worth using. Go buy a fresh bottle.

The Beauty Brains bottom line
Given the importance of good UV protection, don't take chances with a bottle of sunscreen that you think may be bad. Most manufacturers of sunscreen products like Coppertone, Himaya, Ocean Potion, and even Jack Black, should gladly refund your money or offer you a replacement if you have a problem.

Chapter 5
Beauty Biology

Four Types Of Wrinkles And How to Get Rid Of Them

Ellen inquires:

Cosmetics companies don't usually do a good job of explaining the problems they claim to solve. Take anti-wrinkle creams for example. Can someone just please tell me what causes wrinkles in the first place?

The Left Brain Educates:

Since the goal of the Beauty Brains is to educate our community, we thought we'd share the results of a study published in the *International Journal of Cosmetic Science (2006, 28 389-395)*. Researchers at the University

Hospital of Liege, Belgium determined that there actually four distinctly different types of wrinkles that you'll (eventually) have to face.

1. Atrophic Crinkling Rhytids

What they are?

Fine lines on the face that are almost parallel to each other.

Where they occur?

They show up in different areas of the face and body but they tend to disappear when skin is stretched transversally. (that means they shift when your body posture changes.) These wrinkles are associated with loss of elasticity.

What you can do?

Since these wrinkles are due to underlying loss of collagen, you need to protect your skin using sun protectants. You can also use moisturizers to temporarily plump the skin and diminish the appearance of these fine lines.

2. Permanent Elastic Creases

What they are?

These are crease lines in the skin that become increasingly permanent over time, especially with sun exposure.

Where they occur?

They show up most frequently on on the cheek, the upper lip, and the base of the neck.

What you can do?

Sun exposure makes this type of wrinkle worse. So unless you're blessed with naturally dark skin, you should avoid sun exposure or use a sunscreen on these areas to prevent this kind of wrinkling.

3. Dynamic Expression Lines

What they are?

Wrinkles that are caused by facial muscle movement.

Where they occur?

Frown lines and crows feet.

What you can do?

These wrinkles respond to Botox or similar treatments.

4. Gravitational Folds

What they are?

As the name implies, these lines are from the effects of gravity and they become increasingly obvious as skin begins to fold and sag. As we noted in a recent post, skin research on the International Space Station might shed some light on the mechanisms of gravity-induced wrinkles.

Where they occur?

The location of these wrinkles is related to the thickness of skin. While we would have thought this means that thicker skin shows more folds, surprisingly the researchers said that a fat face may show fewer gravity folds than a lean face.

What you can do?

Skin-lifting procedures are effective at removing these kinds of wrinkles.

Unfortunately, wrinkles are a reality of life. Gravity, natural UV radiation and genetics all conspire against us to create them. There is only so much you can do with cosmetics to remove them which is why so many people turn to surgery when they are really desperate. Perhaps the best thing you can do is learn to accept how your body looks. At least until scientists can figure out better solutions.

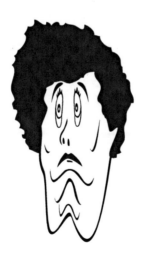

5 Ways To Reduce Enlarged Pores

Jess Just Wants To Know:
I have had large pores for as long as I remember. What products really work to shrink facial pores?

The Right Brain's Reply:
Unfortunately, none. At first glance, you may think that pore control products offer to make your pores smaller, but if you read the label carefully you'll see that in most cases they just claim to reduce the appearance of large pores. That may sound like a subtle distinction but it's really not. There's not much you can do to physically make your pores smaller but you can avoid making them look larger. Instead of looking for "shrinking" products, try avoiding these factors that can make pores look plump:

5 Ways to Reduce Enlarged Pores

1. Skin debris like dead skin cells can collect in pores making them appear bigger. Good facial cleansing is key to staying debris-free.

2. Excessive oiliness can keep pores filled with a layer of oil that accentuates their appearance. Consider using oil-absorbing makeup or more frequent cleansing or blotting.

3. Bacterial growth contribute to blackheads and make pores appear freakishly huge. Exfolliation can help.

4. Sun exposure can thicken the skin cells around the edge of pores making them appear larger. Using a sunscreen or limiting your sun exposure is a good idea.

5. Genetics determines your skin type and if you're unlucky enough to be born with oily, thicker skin your pores will probably be more noticeable. Changing your parents could help this but is probably not a very practical solution.

What Causes Acne?

Lora Longs To Learn About Skintactix and Acne:
As a biophysicist working on her PhD, and as a female, I absolutely LOVE your site. It's such a great way for women to cut through the hype and get some real answers, especially about the products that seem too good to be true.

I have a question about a website I found: www.skintactix.com. This site claims to have a very interesting combination of cleansers in their acne treatment products, and go on to talk very scientifically about how each works to not only kill the bacteria causing acne, but also to stop the process of inflammation at a molecular level. As someone who has struggled with acne since I was a teen, and also someone who is a bit of a dork, the thought intrigued me. Do you think that these ingredients can really stop inflammation, and if so, why don't dermatologists use it?

The Left Brain Talks Types Of Acne:
Lora, thanks for your kind words about The Beauty Brains. Our mission is to educate women about beauty products and we're thrilled that you we can be of help. Now on to your question:

First, you have to realize that there are two kinds of acne: noninflammatory and inflammatory. Second, you have to realize that for acne to occur, 3 conditions must be met:

1. Oil glands gone wild
Your sebaceous glands begin to produce an excessive amount of oil. This increase in oil production is typically, but not always, associated with a change in hormones. That's why teenagers get so many zits, but it can strike adults as well. Either way, the result is that the ducts in your dermis are filled with more oily sebum than usual.

2. Chunky skin is gunky

Your skin cells don't shed properly. Normally your skin cells flake off in very tiny pieces that don't cause any problems. But sometimes they go haywire and start to grow to quickly so they don't flake off properly. When that happens those chunks of cells can mechanically block the outward flow of sebum.

3. Bad bacterial blockage

This is caused the organism Propionibacterium acnes (aka P. acnes) which thrives in the lipid-rich sebum in your oil glands. This bacteria feeds off the oil and grows and grows and grows…

When the first two conditions are met the excess sebum and the dead keratin cells clog your oil duct by forming a follicular plug called a microcomedo. (That's where the term comedogenic comes from, get it?) This tiny plug is the first sign of acne. As more and more gunk fills up the duct, the walls of the hair follicle become swollen and distended. What was a micro comedo now becomes a larger comedo, also known as a whitehead. As the plug continues to grow it starts to poke through the opening of the oil duct and becomes visible as a blackhead. (BTW, Blackheads look black because they contain melanin, the same pigment in your skin that's responsible for your suntan.) Whiteheads and blackheads are technically known as noninflammatory acne.

In inflammatory acne the comedo becomes inflamed and turns into a raised, reddened pus engorged bump. What, you ask, makes the noninflammatory type turn inflammatory? The culprit is lipase, a chemical produced by excessive growth of the P. acnes bacteria. The lipase breaks down the oily triglycerides in your skin, releasing fatty acids. These acids irritate the skin and cause inflammation. (That process has to do with the release of hydrolytic enzymes that break down the follicular wall. But we'll save that story for another post.) Suffice it to say that these acids can turn a simple blackhead into an oozing pus-filled volcano.

So, now that you understand the types of acne and what causes them, we're ready to answer your question about Skintactix. Unfortunately, we're out of time for today so you'll have to return tomorrow to read Part Two. (Aww, I'm such a tease!)

Do Skintactix Ingredients Battle Acne Inflammation

Yesterday we discussed how the bacteria responsible for acne create fatty acids that attack and inflame blackheads. Today we'll finish the discussion and answer Lora's question about dermatologists using ant-inflammatory agents like those in Skintactix.

What's in Skintactix?

This Skintactix line consists primarily of surfactant-based cleansers and exofolliants that use Salicylic Acid as their active ingredient. They also contain a several plant extracts like cinnamon, sage, and thyme. Their website is not exactly clear about the precise purpose of these ingredients, but the implication is that they are anti-inflammatory agents.

Do Skintactix products really work?

Well, Sal acid is an approved anti-acne agent, so I'd expect these products would work as well as similar products on the market. But we can't find any clinical data that suggest the plant extracts they mention have been proven efficacious against acne inflammation.

Anti-inflammatory acne fighters

What about dermatologists? You asked why they don't use anti-inflammatory agents. Well, in reality, they do. The most popularly prescribed anti-acne antibiotics (Tetracycline, Meclocycline, Erythromycin, Clindamycin, Tretinoin) do have anti-inflammatory properties. So when your doctor prescribes this kind of medicine for your zits you're really getting a two-for-one effect: antibiotic and anti-inflammatory. So, if you have a ton of inflamed blackheads, The Beauty Brains think you may need to see your doctor.

How To Pop A Pimple

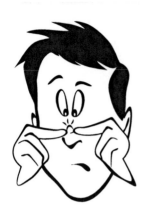

Laurie's concern:
"I have always been told that it's unhealthy and potentially damaging to squeeze my own zits. I'm not Ivanka Trump and I can't afford to hire people to squeeze my pimples on a regular basis. Am I really damaging my skin FOREVER if I pop a pimple? Am I any less qualified to pick at my zits than an esthetician? It doesn't seem like rocket science to me."

The Right Brain's reply:
Our suggestion is to play the Lotto. When you win, you'll be able to hire pimple poppers like the rest of us. In fact, the Left Brain and I use hired help to pop pimples, file warts and, on occasion, lance boils. That's just our way of contributing to the capitalistic culture of cosmetics.

But seriously, by squeezing your own zits you might make them worse. According to the American Academy of Dermatologists, you should NOT pick, scratch, pop, or squeeze pimples yourself because you`ll get more redness, swelling, inflammation, and possible scarring. (If you want to learn more about the causes and effects of acne, read our previous posts.)

But, if you INSIST on throwing caution to the winds and picking those pus pockets yourself, here are some tips:

7 easy steps to popping your own pimples (courtesy of Acne.org.)
1. Take a warm shower or bath to soften your skin.
2. Wash your face and remove all makeup.
3. Wash your hands to prevent spreading germs and infecting the pimple.
4. Sterilize a needle... (a dirty needle will cause an infection and maybe a bigger pimple).
5. Gently prick the tip of the pimple with the needle.

6. Take a clean tissue or piece of toilet paper and wrap it around your index fingers.
7. Gently apply pressure to the sides of the pimple to ease out the pus. Stop when blood or clear fluid comes out.

The Red-faced Regret of Rosacea

Katy has cause for concern:
I have clusters of dry, red raised bumps on either side of my chin. I've been using hydrocortisone that helps but doesn't cure them. I also have a flush to my cheeks and am prone to blushing, which are two characteristics of Rosacea. Does this sound like Rosacea and do you know of any better remedies Hydrocortisone?

The Right Brain rambles on Rosacea:
Katy, based on your description you might have a form of Rosacea but you really should really check with a dermatologist for the best course of treatment. Your question prompted us to include Rosacea in our Cosmetic Diseases and Disorders Series so everyone gains a better understanding of this condition. Hopefully you'll find this information helpful.

What is Rosacea
Rosacea is an inflammatory skin condition that causes the skin around your nose, cheeks, chin and eyes to become very red and flushed. Over 14 million Americans suffer from this neurovascular disorder, according to the National Rosacea Society. Why is this such a disturbing disorder? Because it's more than just a simple case of being red-faced! The condition has psychological effects as well. The Society has done studies that show nearly 70 percent of Rosacea sufferers have lowered self-esteem, and 41 percent say that the condition causes them to avoid public contact or cancel social engagements.

What causes Rosacea?
No one knows for sure but there are several theories. It could be related to how facial blood vessels cope with being flushed and dilated. Or, it could be

that it's an over active inflammatory response to some unknown pathogen. Though the exact cause is unknown, we do know that it can be worsened by harsh skin treatments, strong acne medications, and even exposure to excessive sunlight.

How can you tell if you have Rosacea?
Again, you should consult your dermatologist to find out if your condition really is Rosacea. But here are some common symptoms you can look for. The redness associated with Rosacea primarily occurs in the flushing zone, the nose, cheeks, chin and forehead. Besides the reddening, you may see dilated blood vessels and facial swelling. You may also feel a slight burning sensation on your face. Inflammatory papules and pustules (the red bumps you described?) may develop as well.

You should also note that Rosacea starts as mild episodes of facial blushing or flushing which can turn into a permanently red face over time.

There is a special type of Rosacea, known as Ocular Rosacea, that affects both the eye surface and eyelid. This condition can cause redness, dry eyes, redness, crusting and even loss of eyelashes.

What can you do about Rosacea?
We didn't find any reference to using hydrocortisone to fight Rosacea, but there are other medications that are used to control the redness and reduce the number of papules and pustules.

The most commonly used drugs are oral antibiotics and topical metronidazole. Isotretinoin (Accutane) has also been shown to work against severe papopustular rosacea because it physically shrinks sebaceous glands and it has potent anti-inflammatory properties. And there has been some discussion that topical application of a drug called Finacea may be a promising treatment as well. You'll need a prescription form your doctor for all of these though.

There are some things you can do without a prescription: according to the experts, you should use a gentle cleansing regime to avoid aggravating the condition. So make sure you're using a mild facial cleanser and not scrubbing too much! You should also limit sun exposure by protecting your skin with a good non-irritating sunscreen everyday. You might find a product that uses physical sunblock ingredients like zinc oxide or titanium dioxide might be less aggravating than some of the reactive sunscreens.

For much, much more on this subject, visit the Rosacea Support Group.*

What's The Difference Between Antiperspirant And Deodorant?

Sarah V posts this perspiration puzzle:
What's the difference between an antiperspirant and a deodorant? What gives?

The Right Brain responds:
Sara, thanks for probing this pithy perspiration poser! Here's the real deal: antiperspirants, as the name implies, stop you from perspiring, or sweating. Deodorants simply get rid of odor. Ultimately, both products are trying to do the same thing: stop you from being stinky. But the way they do their deodorizing duty differs.

Why does sweat smell bad?
Before we explain how these products work, let's talk a little bit about perspiration. It works like this: you sweat and bacteria grow in the moist, warm areas where the sweat collects. When the bacteria grow they eat some of the stuff in your sweat (primarily fatty acids) and they poop out stuff that smells bad. End result? B.O. (That's the quick explanation if anyone's interested in the long version, just let us know and we can dedicate a future post to a more detailed discussion on sweat. Or you can read all about it here. And if you're really interested, read this article about how women crave the smell of men's sweat!)

*http://rosacea-support.org/

What do deodorants do?

So, antiperspirants and deodorants offer you two different approaches to fighting smelly bacterial poop. Deodorants contain an active ingredient (Triclosan is most commony used) that prevents the bacteria from growing and devouring your sweat. No bacteria = no body odor. However, you still get Wet Pits (isn't that Brad Pitt's brother?)

How do antiperspirants act?

Antiperspirants, on the other hand, fight the odor problem in a different way. The active ingredients in antiperspirants, typically zinc salts, interact with your sweat glands to stop perspiration. No perspiration = no food for bacteria = no body odor.

Is it bad to plug your pores?

Okay, we know what you're thinking, isn't it bad for you to plug up your sweat glands like that? Don't sweat it. (Ha, that's a pun, get it?) But seriously, it's not something you need to worry about. You're only affecting a small portion of your body's sweat glands so you're not interfering with your body's natural cooling mechanism.

We should also note that antiperspirants do also have some mild anti-bacterial properties, so if you do still sweat little bit not much bacteria will grow. Oh, and by the way, both antiperspirants and deodorants also contain fragrance to cover up any odor that does sneak through.

Wet or dry, how do you decide?

So there you have it two different approaches to solving the same problem. Which one should you use? That's really up to you. Are your arm pits sensitive from shaving? You might want to use a deodorant because some antiperspirants can irritate freshly shaved skin. Do you really, really, really sweat a lot? Then you might need an antiperspirant to avoid dripping. Do you wear black dresses that get white stains from antiperspirants? A clear deodorant might be the way to go.

The Reason Armpit Hair Doesn't Grow Down To Your Knees

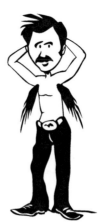

Li Longs To Learn:

How does hair know when to grow? When you shave your legs, it grows back but it stops growing after a certain length. If you shave it again, it will grow back to that length. What's up with that???

The Left Brain Leads Her:

Li, actually your question is easy to answer once you understand two things: the different stages of hair growth and the different kinds of hair your body grows.

Stages of hair growth

The first thing to know is that hair goes through 3 different stages as it grows: Anagen, Catagen and Telogen phases. The Anagen stage (that's Anagen, not Anakin!) is the stage where the hair grows like crazy. This stage can last a up to 4 to 6 years and can produce scalp hairs that grow to be almost 3 feet in length! (that's 100 cm for our international readers). And if you think 3 feet is impressive, you ain't seen nothin'! Human scalp hair longer than 5 feet has been reported! Yikes! We'd hate to see the bill from her stylist!

The Catagen stage follows the Anagen stage. This is basically a transitional stage which means the follicle is slowing down production of the hair, not much happens here.

The third stage is the Telogen, or resting, stage. The hair stops growing and just sits there in the follicle. When the cycle starts all over again with Anagen phase, the old hair is pushed out by the new hair. That's one of the reasons you normally shed about 100 or so hairs each day - the old ones are getting replaced by the new ones.

Types of hairs

The second thing to understand is that there are two different types of hairs: Terminal and Vellus. Terminal are long hairs (the 3 footers we mentioned) and are thicker and have a longer growing cycle (growing season like flowers) 6 to 8 years. Meaning most of the time they are in Anagen phase. These are found on the scalp, mostly. Terminal hairs are the kind you have to cut because they get too long.

Vellus on the other hand are short hairs (a millimeter or less) they are very fine, and they have a very short life cycle, which means they spend most of the time in the Telogen phase. That also means they'll never grow as long as scalp hair. These very fine hairs are found on "hairless" parts of the body like arms and legs. (Ok, those areas aren't hairless, but they kind of look hairless because the hairs are so tiny and fine.)

Soooo, to answer your question, that's how hair knows when to grow - it's determined by the type of hair and the stage of growth it's in. Which of course is determined by hormones. Isn't everything?

Top 5 Causes of Darkened Armpits

Germaine Pie Is Puzzled By Her Pits:
What causes darkened armpits and what can we do to get rid of them?
They're so embarrassing!

The Right Brain Raises Her From the Pit of Despair:
It's not surprising that so many people have this problem - there are
at least FIVE different reasons your pits could be darker than they should be.

1. Shaving
When you shave you cut the hairs off at, or just below, the surface of the skin.
If your hairs are slightly darker than your skin color, they can give the appearance
that your skin has a dark stain when it's really just sub-surface hair.

What To Do About It:
Stop shaving and try waxing or plucking instead so you get rid of the hair below
the skin surface. Since the hairs aren't lurking so close to the top of your skin,
they won't be as visible.

2. Buildup of dead skin cells
According to at least one dermatolgist, dark spots under your arms are the result
of dead skin cells that are trapped in microscopic "hills and valleys" on your
skin.

What To Do About It:
Exfoliate, preferably with a product containing lactic acid.

3. Antiperspirant and deodorant usage
In theory, some ingredients in these products (perhaps the fragrance) could be
reacting with the skin to cause discoloration. Practically speaking this seems
unlikely but many people do claim that when they stop using APDs, the darkness
goes away.

What To Do About It:
Try switching brands or using a deodorant instead of an antiperspirant. You
may stink a bit more, but hey, the Left Brain lives for experiments like that!

4. A medical condition called acanthosis nigricans
This condition causes light-brown-to-black markings on the neck, under the
arms, or in the groin. It can be related to insulin production or to a glandular
disorder and it typically occurs in people who are overweight.

- continued on next page

What To Do About It:
Watch your diet to control insulin production and use Retin A, 20% urea, alpha hydroxyacids, and salicylic acid prescriptions to lighten your armpits.

5. Hyper-pigmentation
This condition causes your skin to produce excess melanin pigment. It doesn`t usually affect armpits, so it's a less likely cause.

What To Do About It:
Use a skin bleaching cream to destroy the excess melanin. The Beauty Brains don't recommend this unless you consult a dermatologist first. You can also try laser treatment to destroy the pigment.

How To Tell The Difference Between Skin Irritation and Skin Allergy

Grace is grumbling:
I have severe allergies to dust and pollen and it really bugs me when I hear my friends say they're "allergic" to cosmetics. I don't think they're allergic, the cosmetics are probably just irritating their skin. Please tell me who's right so I can make them shut up!

The Right Brain Has An Allergic Response:
Actually you AND your friends might be right. Certain cosmetic chemicals can cause negative reactions in some people. There are two basic types of reactions: irritation reaction (also known as Irritant Contact Dermatitis, or ICD) and allergic response (known as Allergic Contact Dermatitis or ACD). In general terms, irritation occurs when your cells are attacked by harsh chemicals. An allergy occurs when your immune system develops antibodies in response to a chemical you've been exposed to. (Just like your hayfever.)

It's important to understand if you're irritated or allergic because it will help your doctor determine the right course of treatment. Here's how you can tell the difference.

What They Do To Your Skin

Irritation: Gives you redness with possible oozing sores. Your skin may develop a chapped, glazed or scaled appearance. You'll feel burning, stinging, pain and soreness. You may also have some itchiness.

Allergies:

The skin appearance may be similar, but the main symptom is itchiness.

Where The Response Occurs

Irritation: The effects are usually limited to the part of the skin that was contacted by the chemical.

Allergy: Because you're producing antibodies, the effect is not limited to the contact point. The effects may be worse in the contact area, but you can develop symptoms any where on your body.

How Long It Takes For The Response To Develop

Irritation: Symptoms develop after a single exposure. They usually appear in a few minutes, at most within a few hours, after contact.

Allergies: After the first exposure, you typically have no symptoms. That's because your body hasn't developed an antibody response to the agent yet. After subsequent exposures, Symptoms may take 24 to 72 hours to develop.

Source: *Dermatotoxicology, 6th edition. Edited by Hongbo Zhai and Howard I. Maibach*

Chapter 6
Marvelous Makeup

Are You Addicted To Lip Balm?

Chris is Curious:
Is it really possible to be addicted to lip balm?

The Left Beauty Brain's Lips Respond:
Fascinating question, Chris. And you can find an equally fascinating, but a little over-analyzed, discussion on the addictive properties of lip balm at Lip Balm Anonymous. The post is a bit outdated but we found it to be an interesting reference, nonetheless.

But the one argument that we did NOT see discussed was, in our opinion, the most scientifically valid one. It goes something like this:

Skin signals for new cells

Skin is a very complicated organ with multiple layers. The top layer, the stratum corneum, consists mainly of dead, dried up cells. As those cells die and flake off, they send a signal to a deeper layer skin (called the basal layer) to produce fresh skin cells. This is a very simplified description of the process called cellular turnover. (Contrary to what you might have thought, "cellular turnover" does NOT refer to switching your mobile phone plan.)

Lip balm slows down the signal

When you apply lip balm, you're creating a barrier layer that prevents, or at least retards, the evaporation of moisture from the inner layers of skin. Since the top layer isn't drying and flaking off as much, the basal layer never gets the signal to produce new cells.

Your skin has to catch up

But when you stop using the lip balm, all of a sudden your lips dry out and your basal layer has to hurry up and start producing new cells. But since your lips already feel dry again, you add more lip balm which once again tells the basal layer "hey, everything's fine up here on the surface - we don't need any more new skin cells."

The cycle repeats

But of course, once that application of lip balm has worn off and there are no new plump, moist skin cells to replace the ones that are drying out, your lips feel dry again and you have to add more lip balm. Etc. etc. etc. Get the picture? That's why you feel addicted to lip balm - you've "trained" you body to rely on it!

This theory provides a more scientific explanation for the mysterious Lip Balm Addiction and it seems to make sense for most balm users.

Do Eye Creams Really Work?

Lucy Longingly Asks:
I just bought Eyecon from Benefit, but I'm not sure if it's really doing anything. What are eye creams and is their claim of reducing under eye circles and puffiness at all valid? What ingredients should I look for in an eye cream for these things?

The Right Brain Strikes An Optic Nerve:
Do eye creams really do what they say they'll do? Well, the answer is a little bit yes, a little bit no. All skin creams (should) moisturize. But eye creams have some added responsibilities.

1. Moisturization
They've got to moisturize without adding a lot of heaviness or greasiness. After all, it's likely that you'll be apply some kind of make up around your eyes and you don't want an eye cream to interfere with your foundation, for example.

2. Mildness
They need to be extra mild, since the area around the eye is particularly sensitive to irritation. Fragrance free is best.

3. Tightening
Perhaps most relevant to your question, they should tighten the skin around the eyes since they claim to reduce wrinkles. While they can't work miracles, they can do this to some extent by adding polymers that form a film on the skin as they dry. This film can make the skin look and feel a little bit tighter.

The Eyecon product you cited seems designed to do just that. It contains ingredients like Ethylene/Acrylic Acid Copolymer, Butylene Glycol, Glyceryl Polymethacrylate, and Sodium Polyacrylate. These are all film forming agents that can help eyes feel less puffy and look less wrinkled.

Of course the effect varies from person to person; even in best case scenarios it may not be dramatically noticible; and even if it does work it's only a temporary fix at best. But if you notice enough difference you might want to continue using the product.

Want another opinion? Paula Begoun, the Cosmetic Cop, has a much harsher opinion of eye creams. She says that they are no different from facial moisturizers and that they are "a whim of the cosmetics industry designed to evoke the sale of two products when only one is needed." Meow!

The Beauty Brains bottom line

Eye creams are essentially moisturizers that are modified for use on the thin skin around the eyes. While they don't work miracles like they claim, they do contain ingredients that may offer some temporary benefit. We say: try it and see what you think. But as always, let the buyer beware.

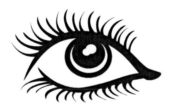

Do Lip Plumpers Really Work?

Jessie Just Wants To Know:
I recently tried a lip plumper while browsing in Sephora. I was skeptical, but then as I walked around the store, I really did notice my lips feeling slightly fuller and very tingly. Is this my imagination? What are lip plumpers and how do they work?

The Right Brain Responds:
Lip plumpers work by temporarily irritating lips and causing them to swell slightly. That tingly feeling is not your imagination, it's your lips reacting to a menthol type chemical that most plumpers use. The effect is slight and temporary - don't expect to look like you've had a collagen injection. And while these products really do have this effect, the bad news it's not really good for your lips to use them on a regular basis because it can be damaging to the skin.

Look for menthoxypropanediol on the ingredient list if you're not sure the product will really plump or not.

Why Smashbox Should Be Ashamed of O-Glow Blush

Tamara's Intrigued:
Smashbox's O-Glow gel claims to generate a natural blushing effect by stimulating skin circulation. I'm intrigued, but the thought of intentionally inflaming my cheeks with a foreign substance strikes me as a bit weird. Does this really work?

The Right Brain Blushes:
Let's take a look, shall we? According to Smashbox: "This revolutionary silicone-based clear gel works on every skin tone and is microcirculating and skin energizing to keep cheeks naturally flushed for hours." O-Glow

does change to a pink color, but not for the reasons Smashbox gives us. We captured our evaluation of this product in the following pictures:

Every picture tells a story
If you follow the link to our blog (http://thebeautybrains.com/2007/07/10/ why-smashbox-should-be-ashamed-of-o-glow-blush) you'll see three pictures that tell O-blush story. The first one shows that O-Glow is a clear, colorless gel when it comes out of the tube. The second shows that when rubbed on your cheek, it does turn from colorless to a lovely shade of pink. But is a "micro-circulatory effect" really causing the color? The third picture has the answer: the product changes color even when it's applied to a piece of white paper. Since paper doesn't have blood vessels, it's obvious that the effect has nothing to do with the circulatory system.

How does it really work?
So how does it change color? Could it be the Red Dye #27 that's listed as one of the ingredients? Yep. I'll spare you the gory chemical details but essentially the red dye is colorless when dissolved in a waterless base. When it comes in contact with moisture, the change in solubility and pH causes the dye to turn bright pink. That moisture can come from your skin, or even just the humidity in the air. So really, this product uses a dye to stain your cheeks just like any other blush.

The Beauty Brains bottom line
While we appreciate the clever formulation work required to make a color changing product, we say shame on Smashbox for presenting it in such a misleading way. It's a cool gimmick, but this product does NOT do what they say it does. Considering how they're blatantly lying to us about this blush, Smashbox should be the ones with the red face!

Do You Believe The Promise Of Lip Gloss That Helps You Lose Weight?

A while back we reported a story about how a fragrance can make it look like you've lost weight. Well, Omega Tech Labs has introduced a lip gloss called Promise that is supposed to have weight loss benefits.

Appetite suppressant in lip gloss

According to the company, the lip gloss contains a blend of botanical oils (castor oil, coconut oil and evening primrose oil) that work as appetite suppressants. Experts say that these ingredients can work but they don't believe you will get enough exposure from the lip gloss to make much difference.

Smells can help you slim

While this Beauty Brain is highly skeptical, there is some science backing up the product concept. Researchers at the Smell & Taste Treatment and Research Foundation have done studies showing that odors can actually help people lose Marvelous Makeup weight. If Promise lip gloss contains appetite suppressant oils and odors that help curb your appetite, it might have an effect.

Could be too tasty

On the other hand, the flavor could actually stimulate your appetite and have the opposite effect! Since the company offers no clinical study, we can't know for sure whether it works. But it's probably worth a try. It will certainly be a good lip gloss and if it has the added benefit of helping you lose weight without taking another spinning class, how cool is that?

How Mascara Makes Lashes Look Lovely

We've had several readers ask how mascara is made and how it works, so here's the sciencey scoop:

History of mascara

First a quick bit of background - we know that mascaras have been around since at least 4000 BC because historical records show that Egyptians used charcoal and other minerals to darken their lashes and eyelids. In modern times, mascara first appeared in the form of a pressed cake that was applied by wetting a brush, rubbing it on the cake, and than applying it to eye lashes. The cake consisted of a mixture of black pigments and soap chips. The next innovation in mascara involved a lotion like version of the soap cake that was packaged in a tube and squeezed onto a small brush to apply. Mascara as we know it today was created in the 1960s with the invention of a grooved brush that could apply a consistent amount. This is the basic form that's still used today.

Common ingredients

The primary ingredients in mascara are pigments - the chemicals that provide color. Because U.S. Federal regulations only allow certain colorants to be used in area of the eye, only natural colors and inorganic pigments are used. Carbon black and iron oxides provide black, brown , and red colors; chemicals Ultramarine blue provide blue and green shades. Manufacturing, Mixing, and Packaging: These pigments are mixed together in a cosmetic base that is an emulsion of oils , waxes, and water. For examples of these waxy ingredients, let's look at an example formulation from Maybelline Great Lash:

Water, Beeswax, Ozokerite, Shellac, Glyceryl Stearate, Triethanolamine, Propylene Glycol, Stearic Acid, Sorbitan Sesquioleate, Methylparaben, Quaternium-15, Quaternium-22, Simethicone, Butylparaben, Iron Oxides (may contain), Titanium Dioxide (may contain), Ultramarine Blue

The Beeswax, Ozokerite, Stearic Acid, and Shellac provide the main body of the mascara and give it it's waterproof and smudge proof properties. Glyceryl Stearate and Triethanolamine are added to make sure the mascara can be washed off. The Propylene Glycol, Sorbitan Sesquioleate, and Simethicone, added as processing agents and help control the consistency of the product while Methylparaben, Quaternium-15, Quaternium-22, and Butylparaben are preservatives that keep the mascara free of "bugs" Finally, the Iron Oxides Titanium Dioxide Ultramarine Blue are the pigments.

How mascara is made

These ingredients are mixed together in large metal kettles. Typically, the waxes and emulsifiers are mixed together and melted in one vessel and the water soluble ingredients are mixed in another vessel. Once the waxes are completely melted, the pigments are added. When both portions are sufficiently heated and mixed , they are blended together to form the final product. A device known as a homogenizer is used to make sure all the pigment particles are properly dispersed. Once the mascara is finished mixing, it is transferred to a filling machine that pumps a metered amount into each glass or plastic mascara bottle. The brush or wand is inserted into the tube and a capping machine automatically twists it shut. The tubes are then packaged for shipping.

How mascara works

This is really the simple part - when you stick the brush into the mascara tube and pull it out, a metering ring built into the orifice scrapes off the excess mascara so the brush has a controlled dose on it. So, when you brush your eye lashes, just the right amount gets delivered to each tiny hair fiber. The waxy nature of the mascara helps form a relatively thick coating that, due to the high wax concentration, is very water proof. That's how a good mascara can resist smudging and bleeding. The result - your eye lashes get a nice splash of color and they look much plumper.

Is Your Lip Plumper Making You Sick?

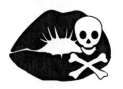

Melanie is miserable:
Recently, I had a terrible allergic reaction on my lips to the Primal Elements Lip Plumper. Shortly after putting it on I had severe swelling, bumps, peeling, on and on. My dermatologist prescribed cortisone cream that seems to be working it will be awhile until it's completely healed. Do you have an idea of what could have caused a reaction. Maybe the cinnamon? Do you have any suggestions about lip balms that will be safe to use in the future.

The Left Brain provides lip service:
We've written about lip plumpers before, so I looked at the ingredient list of this product and have some theories about which ingredients might be the problem.

Spicy hot?
First, you asked about cinnamon. That's a good guess because Cinnamic aldehyde, a component of cinnamon oil, is known to cause allergy contact dermatitis. Symptoms include a rash, intense swelling, and redness of the affected area.

However, that doesn't seem to be the likely culprit for your lip gloss because Primal Elements doesn't contain cinnamon oil, it contains Ethylhexyl Methoxycinnamate which is a sunscreen. While the name sounds like cinnamon, it's not. Some people are sensitive to sunscreens, however, so you could look at the ingredients on other products you buy and see if you've used this one before.

Icky irritants?
What else? Well, Menthol and Camphor are mild irritants that could be causing the problem. And Benzyl Nicotinate is added to give your lips the tingling feeling that lip plumpers are supposed to provide. You might be reacting to that.

Smells like fragrance

Finally, fragrance is always one of the usual suspects when it comes to skin reactions. The good news is, probably any lip gloss you try will have a different fragrance than Primal Elements. The rest of the formula seems unlikely to cause a problem.

The Beauty Brains bottom line:

If you look for a lip gloss that doesn't have ethyl methoxycinnamate, menthol, camphor, benzyl nicotinate and that has a different fragrance, that should help.

Does Blinc Kiss Me Mascara Work

Amy Asks:

I have recently purchased Blinc's Kiss Me Mascara. It works, via their product description, as "tubing" your lashes instead of "painting" them. Let me tell you, it's beyond cool to take of my mascara at night and physically see it coming off in tubes from just "water and pressure" as the directions advise. My eyes water when it's cold out, so I've found that my standard mascara doesn't work in frigid temperatures. I've resorted to a fiber mascara, but I do like this tubing since it is easier to take this off. Can you explain how it works?...Like a good reader, I do know how "standard" mascara works.

The Right Brain Answers:

Hairspray in a mascara

Unlike most mascaras which are made with waxes, Blinc's Kiss Me is formulated with acrylate polymers. These polymers are similar to the ones used in hairsprays and they're what give Kiss Me its ability to form tiny tubes.

Two kinds of strength

When you apply any mascara to your lashes you're coating the tiny hairs with a layer of product. When you try to remove the mascara, two factors come into play: cohesive strength (how well the mascara sticks to itself) and adhesive strength (how well it sticks to the eyelash.)

The coolness of Blinc

Regular mascaras, even LashFusion, have a low cohesive strength and a relatively high adhesive strength. That means when you try to remove regular mascaras they come off in little bits and pieces. Kiss Me mascara, on the other hand, has a high cohesive strength and lower adhesive strength. Therefore, the mascara tends to stay in one piece as it slides off your lashes. That's why it looks like tiny tubes. That is cool!

Science and St. Valentines Day - The Color Of Love

The color RED has long been associated with St. Valentine's Day. It's the color of the blood the runs through our hearts so it's not surprising it's always been linked to love and passion. So today we're blogging about where red dye comes from.

We see the color of passion reflected all over fashion and cosmetics. Everyone has (or should have!) a sexy red lipstick or nail polish for special romantic occasions. (Revlon's Poppysilk Red Lipstick and OPI`s I`m Not Really A Waitress nail polish come to mind.) These products and many others exist thanks to the miracle of modern chemistry which has given us colorants such as FD&C Red No. 40 and D&C Red No. 33.

Of course, we weren't always lucky enough to have such a rainbow of reds to choose from. Originally red dye came from a more natural, yet more disgusting, source: crushed insect bodies. The cochineal insect be precise.

Red Dye From Dead Bugs

These bugs grow in certain varieties of cacti. They're hand picked and immersed in hot water to kill them and to dissolve waxy coating of their shells. The dead bugs are dried in the sun and then ground into a fine powder that can used as dye for fabrics, foods, and cosmetics.

Today, modern chemistry can synthetically create a wide variety of red dyes so we don't have to rely on picking bugs off cacti to make our pucker look pretty. And that's just one more reason to be thankful for cosmetic chemists!

Jan Marini Admits It - Age Intervention Eyelash Product Does Not Grow Hair

One of the most popular topics on the Beauty Brains is the Jan Marini Age Intervention Eyelash. People always want to know, "will this product make my eyelashes grow?" "Is it worth $160 for less than 1 ounce of product?"

No evidence for lash growth

We've looked high and low but have not been able to find any scientific studies that would support that this product will make your eyelashes grow thicker and longer. But that hasn't stopped people from leaving comments telling us how wrong we are. They insist that there is a special off-label glaucoma drug that Jan Marini uses in the product to make eyelashes grow. Or they insist that they've used it and it makes their eyelashes grow. While we're skeptical, we continue to look for credible research that shows this product really works.

Passionate comments

Here is a recent comment that prompted some more research. Jim writes...

Everyone has a right to their opinion, but blatant misinformation is not only inaccurate, but harmful. The new Age Intervention Eyelash product does work. Jan

Marini Skin Research replaced the original prostaglandin analog with another customized prostaglandin analog that actually appears to be even more effective than the original. There was never a patent issue and Jan Marini Skin Research has patents pending on both the original and new formulations. The product has enormous positive media attention along with a huge celebrity following. Physicians throughout the US and abroad have validated the tremendous efficacy of the formula and continue to recommend it to their patients. There is no doubt regarding the amazing results. In addition, the company has excellent safety studies. This continued bashing and misinformation needs to stop. A loyal and informed fan.

Patent pending?

Well, there are certainly some testable claims here even though no references were given. First, we looked at the claim that they've got patents pending. Well, a search at the United States Patent Office reveals no such patents pending for Jan Marini.

Second, "the product does work." This we agree with. Jan Marini Age Intervention Eyelash does work, just like every other mascara you can buy. It DOES NOT work to make your eyelashes grow longer or thicker and we have excellent proof.

What does Jan Marini say?

Just look at what the company says on their own website about the Age Intervention product. We quote

"Age Intervention Eyelash Conditioner is not intended to stop, prevent, cure, relieve, reverse or reduce eyelash loss or to promote the growth of eyelashes"

The company admits that it will not grow your eyelashes! What more proof is needed?

Word of mouth

Third, that a product has a "huge celebrity following" and is endorsed by unnamed physicians throughout the US is not proof of anything. Everyone is susceptible to glitzy marketing and wishful thinking. And if you've spent $160 for a cosmetic to make your eyelashes grow, you probably don't want to admit that you've been fooled. It's ok, no one wants to but it happens.

How Does Eyeliner Work?

The authors of some of the other beauty blogs have asked us to explain how eyeliner works. So here's how 'liners make you lovely!

Types of Eyeliners
Eyeliners are formulated into two basic types: pencils and liquids. While the details vary, both types use these same basic ingredients.

Basic Ingredients
The Base is the backbone of the formula. In the case of pencils, its the waxy/greasy matrix that forms the core of the pencil; in the liquids its the water/oil emulsion in which the rest of the ingredients are suspended.

Typical base ingredients include waxes and oils, emollients (spreading agents) and in the case of liquid type, water and emulsifiers.

Colors
Colorants used in eyeliners (and other cosmetics used around the eye) must be approved by the FDA (in the United States). Colorants that can be used in products for other parts of the body aren't necessarily safe enough to be used around your eyes.

Typical colorants include iron oxides and ultramarine pigments. Carmine is another colorant you see from time to time. It's a red color made from crushed insect bodies. Mmmmm!

Control agents

These are added to eyeliner formulations to make sure the product meets specifications when it's manufactured and that it maintains high quality afer manufacture. These include chemicals that control the pH, or acid/base balance of the product, and that keep the product free of bacteria and mold. In some oil based formulas, an antioxidant may be added to keep the waxes and oils from going rancid.

Typical control agents include tocopherol (also known as vitamin E) used for its antioxidant properties as well as Citric Acid, Methylparaben, and Propylparaben.

Featured ingredients

Several things can be added to eyeliners to make them more appealing to consumers. These ingredients don't change the way the product works or the way it looks, but marketers add them because women think they are helpful.

For some reason aloe vera is a very typical featured ingredient.

Now you know, what next?

There are two ways that understanding eyeliner ingredients could be helpful. Let's say your favorite eyeliner is being discontinued. If you know what kind of base ingredients to look for, you might be able to pick a replacement without having to try so many new products.

On the flip side, if you're getting irritation or an allergic reaction to your eyeliner, you might be able to figure out what ingredients to stay away from when you shop for a new one.

Why Does My Foundation Make My Skin Photograph White?

Karina's Question:

Could you please tell me what the ingredient is in foundation that makes your face look much whiter in photos?!?! Is it just one ingredient, or a combination? Could you recommend any brands which don't do this? Thanks.

The Right Brain Responds:

Karina, we've never heard of this problem before, but we can make an educated guess about what's happening.

Flashback from sunblock

One common ingredient in foundations is titanium dioxide. It's very opaque and so it's good at concealing skin flaws. But it's also good at scattering light rays. In fact, it's used as a sunblock for this very reason. (For example, Neutrogena Healthy Skin Liquid Make up contains 2% titanium dioxide.)

So, our guess is that the brand you're using has more titanium dioxide that's reflecting a lot of white light which shows up in your photographs. Of course, it's also possible that talc or one of the other white powders in the formula could be causing the problem too. There's no way to be sure without testing.

The Beauty Brains bottom line

It's just a guess, but you could try looking for foundations that do NOT have titanium dioxide on the ingredient list. We can't recommend any specific brands, but you can check the ingredients on Drugstore.com.

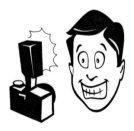

Scientific Proof That Make-up Really Helps

Many women spend countless hours a year putting on cosmetics and making sure they look just right before going out. Did you ever wonder if it was all worth it? Is the make-up really making you look that much more attractive? According to a team of psychologists out of the UK, it is.

In their study, they found that men are more attracted to women with more coloring on their face. And they suggest that there is a good biological basis for this fact. They theorize that women with higher levels of estrogen naturally have more color than those with lower levels. And a higher level of estrogen is indicative of a more fertile woman. According to evolutionary theory, men should be inclined to find more fertile women more attractive.

Marvelous Makeup
The experiment involved measuring hormone levels of a group of volunteer women and then having those women rated for attractiveness by another group of both men and women. It turns out that the ones who were rated highest in attractiveness were also the ones who had the highest level of estrogen.

The Beauty Brains bottom line
Of course, you probably didn't need a scientific study to validate the use of make-up. People discovered the benefits centuries ago. But we here at the Beauty Brains are happy to know that it really isn't all just a waste of time. And it's also nice to know that the chosen career of this Brain is playing a crucial role in the noble quest of successfully propagating a diverse population.

Rouge on people, rouge on.

Do You Make This Major Make Up Mistake?

Sandy Says:
On the back of my daily cleanser (Alpha Hydrox Nourishing Cleanser to be specific) it instructs to apply with an "upward motion". Is there any actual reason for this, or was it just thrown in to seem more "special"? Should I be applying other products in a certain direction/motion?

The Right Brain Responds:
We aren't aware of any real scientific need to apply facial cleansers with an upward motion. Our guess is that it's marketing speak to make the product sound more special. Maybe they think that since gravity drags your skin down (making it saggy and wrinkled) you can push your skin up to get rid of wrinkles. Who knows what they really mean.

How You Apply Cosmetics Can Make A Difference
Does your application technique ever make a difference? Yes, in some cases it does. Sunscreens, for example, need to be applied with very even, smooth strokes because they won't work very well if they don't evenly coat the skin. Same thing is true for sunless tanners if you don't apply them consistently you'll end up with streaks. Some types of make up have similar application issues you need to be careful when applying wrinkle concealing foundations to make sure they fill in those fine lines evenly.

The Beauty Brains bottom line
For some products, application technique does make a difference. That's not the case for facial cleansers. Whether it be Avotone or StriVectin, there's no technical reason that applying the product this way should help your skin. On the other hand, it won't hurt it either.

What Does Borax Do In Lush Lip Balms?

Debby, from the Lush Forum, asks this question:
There has been a discussion about the use of Sodium Borate in some of the lip balms from Lush. Could you tell us something more about this ingredient?

The Right Brain Replies:
Thanks for the question Debby. A lot of people ask us if Lush formulas are really different than mass market products. In this case, they are.

What is Borax?
Sodium Borate, also called Borax, is used in products that contain high levels of beeswax. The Borax reacts with the beeswax to form an emulsion, a stable mixture of oil and water.

How is Lush different than regular products?
Most emulsions, like your typical skin lotion, are "oil in water" emulsions which means that the oil drops are dispersed in the water. Borax-beeswax emulsions are unusual - they're "water in oil" emulsions so the water drops are dispersed in the oil. That type of emulsion tends to be more water proof which is good for a lip balm. Also, because the borax - beeswax combination forms a stable emulsion without the help of additional emulsifiers, this type of formula supports Lush's position of not using excessive chemicals.

Is Borax safe?
And a final note: if you do any kind of web search on Borax you'll find that it can also be used as an insecticide, but don't worry about that. It's only toxic to humans at very high levels - in fact it has the same toxicity profile as common table salt. (Hey, even water can be toxic if you drown in the stuff!) So a little bit in your lip balm is perfectly fine.

Chapter 7
Nail Knowledge You Need

Don't Get Ripped Off By Your Nail Salon

Jennifer's Jittery:
My nail salon uses a UV nail polish dryer. Should I be worried about age spots on the top of my hands and feet from the UV light?

The Right Brain enlightens her:
We looked into UV dryers and found that the wavelength of the light they produce IS the same type that causes photo-aging and skin cancer. (That's the UVA range from about 320 nm to 400 nm for those of you keeping score at home.)

Nail dryers won't cause sunburn

Fortunately, the danger seems pretty slight because drying lamps have a very low power output, only around 10 watts. Compare that to the power of a full sized tanning bed that can put out up to 2400 watts! So your fingers probably aren't in much danger. Still, if you're concerned you could apply some sunblock before using the lamp.

(Are any of you nail salon owners out there listening? That would be a great way to plus up your service for your customers. Offer them a little sunscreen to moisturize and protect the skin of their fingers while the nail lamp is doing its drying duty.)

But they can still be dangerous

So is there ANY danger associated with using UV drying lamps? Yes, in fact, you might be in danger of getting ripped off!

That's because UV light only works on special, more expensive, topcoats that contain a certain type of acrylic polymer that is cross linked by the light. Some salons try to save money by using a regular top coat before using the drying lamp. The UV light won't do anything to make that kind of polish dry faster. So whether you use OPI, Sally Hansen, or any other brand, it makes sense to ask what top coat the nail technician is using so you can make sure you're getting what you pay for!

Four Easy Tips For Longer, Stonger Nails

Webmaster Wants To Know:
I've stopped biting my nails and now I'm trying to grow them out. However, after they reach a certain length they would start to break. I've been using Sally Hansen Hard as Nails, but to no avail! Therefore, my question are: Are the ingredients in Sally Hansen more harmful than helpful to growing my nails and possible health? Are there any nail products that you could recommend that could promote stronger nails?

The Right Brain responds:
The idea that nail hardeners can help your nails grow longer is a myth; but here are four things you CAN do to help your nails:

1. Avoid nail polishes containing formaldehyde.
This chemical can cross link the keratin protein in your nails. While it does make the nails harder, it also makes them so stiff that they become brittle so they actually break MORE easily.

2. Don't bother with gelatin.
Many products claim that gelatin strengthens nails because it is made from protein, but there is no scientific evidence that gelatin has any benefit to nails.

3. Limit your use of polish removers.
These products contain alcohol and other solvents that dry nails out, making them more prone to breakage.

4. Use a good hand cream or cuticle cream.
Daily exposure to detergents and harsh chemicals dries out your nails and makes them break more easily. By moisturizing them often you can prevent loss of moisture and reduce the chance of breakage. Lotions with petrolatum or mineral oil are the best. You might try the Terra Naturals Nail Strengthener.

Source: American Academy of Dermatologists, 10/06

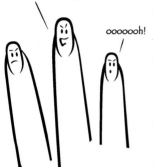

So, me and da' other fingers ...
we're not likin' some of yer habits.
Der better be changes ... or else!!

ooooooh!

Five Ways To Ruin Your Finger Nails

Debby's in Digit Danger:

My fingernails go through seasonal cycles. Sometimes they are long, strong and healthy. At other times, like right now, they split and bend and look ragged. I've used Sally Hansen's Maximum Growth, but it doesn't seem to do much. Got any ideas? Also, why does Sally Hansen have so many products that all seem to do the same thing (i.e., Hard As Nails, Maximum Growth, etc.)?

The Right Brain Hammers Out A Reply For Her Nails:
It's hard to say for sure what the seasonal changes are that you're experiencing, but many things can affect the condition of your nails. Here's our top 5 finger factors to avoid when your nails look hammered.

1. Excessive environmental dryness

Are your nails worse in the winter? If your nail condition is literally changing with the seasons, it may be due to humidity. Nails, like skin, are subject to the drying effects of the environment. Solution: If your nails are dry and raggedy in the winter use more lotion.

2. Hyper hand washing

Does your job (or hobby or home life) cause you to wash your hands on some occasions more than others? Washing your hands with soap and water can dry out nails. That could be causing an apparent seasonal change. Solution: Use a mild hand wash instead of bar soap and don't skimp on the lotion.

3. Damage from drying solvents

Are you engaged in any activities that would expose your nails to solvents? For example, home repair projects (like painting a room or varnishing wood trim) could be seasonal activites that negatively impact the condition of your nails. Solution: make your husband do it. (That's a suggestion from Sarah.)

4. Negative nail product usage

Do you occasionally use nail hardening products? Since you asked about several Sally Hansen products, I'm guessing you do. Those products do make nails harder but they can also make them brittle and more prone to breaking. That's because they use a chemical called formaldehyde to cross link the keratin protein in nails. Solution: Skip the hardeners and see if it helps. (And to answer your question about why they have so many products that seem to do the same thing, we have one word: Capitalism.)

5. The horrible heartbreak of psoriasis

Psoriasis is a disease that causes your skin to become red and scaly. About half the people who suffer from this condition also have nail problems, particularly pitting, rippling, and/or splitting of the nail. Unfortunately, there is no cure for psoriasis, so you'll have to amputate the affected fingers. (Just kidding; I wanted to see if you were still reading.) Solution: If you think psoriasis might be responsible for your nail problems, check with a dermatologist for treatment options.

Is Nail Polish Bad To Breathe?

Laura breathes this question:
Is inhaling nail polish fumes harmful if you're exposed to them for about 30 minutes or so per week?

The Left Brain exhales this response:
Nearly all the popular brands of nail polishes including Revlon and OPI contain organic solvents and methacrylates. The March 2002 issue of Neuropsychiatry, Neuropsychology, & Behavioral Neurology summarizes a study by Gina LaoSasso, Ph.D et.al, that shows prolonged exposure to nail polish fumes can affect the way your brain works.

The researchers tested 33 nail-salon technicians compared to the same number of demographically similar control subjects (in other words, women who had no exposure to nail polish or other toxic chemicals.) Both groups were given a series of psychologic, neuropsychologic, and neurosensory tests.

Nail Polish Fumes Affect Brain Functions

Their study showed three main results:
1. The nail technicians performed statistically worse than the control group on tests that measured attention and brain processing speed.
2. The nail technicians and the control group showed no statistical differences in learning and memory, fine motor coordination, or on measures of depression and anxiety.
3. The nail technicians' sense of smell was statistically worse than the control group's.

Fresh air, not fumes
What does all this mean? Apparently, exposure to enough nail polish fumes can make your brain a little slow and fuzzy. Kinda scary, huh? Unfortunately, the study didn't provide details on how long this effect lasts so we don't know if your brain returns to normal once you've gotten away from the nail fumes.

And while the study did measure the size of the salon, the amount of ventilation, and the number of hours that the technicians worked, the data can't be used to predict what would happen at a lower exposure. In other words, if you're in a nail salon long enough, you may experience these problems. But is 30 minutes a week enough to cause an effect? It doesn't look like it but clearly more studies are needed. In the meantime, make sure you're getting plenty of fresh air when you're getting your nails done!

Color, not die!
Note if you happened to be talking about inhaling the fumes on purpose

(huffing) we would strongly advise against this. According to this article about huffing

"Death from inhalant abuse can occur after a single use or after prolonged use. Sudden sniffing death (SSD) may result within minutes of inhalant abuse from irregular heart rhythm leading to heart failure."

Now, it's not very likely that you will die but it's certainly not worth the risk.

Why Does Wearing Polish Turn My Nails Yellow?

Sue Says:
I was wondering why does wearing nail polish turn your nails yellow? Also, is there anything we can do to prevent that?

The Right Brain Polishes Off This Response:
Nail polish can turn your nails yellow. Why? There are a couple of reasons:

Color reaction
Some of the darker colored polishes can stain nails due to a chemical reaction between the colorant and the nail plate. This reaction is hard to predict because it doesn't happen for everybody for every dark color. It can also take a few days to a few weeks to occur.

Formaldehyde
It's also possible that formaldehyde (one of the ingredients in many nail polishes) is causing the problem. This chemical can react with the keratin protein in your nails and make it brittle and yellow.

Medical issues

Finally, if your nails are really yellowed and disfigured, you may have a nail infection or a more serious medical condition known as Yellow Nail Syndrome. So what can you do about it? Read on!

Tips for non-yellowing nails

1. Don't try to scrape off the stained area because it will damage and weaken the nail.
2. Stay away from dark colors (which will greatly reduce your fashion options)
3. Wear a base coat to protect your nails from staining (this makes sense to us)
4. Look for nail polishes that don't have formaldehyde on the ingredient list. (There's no guartentee that this will work but hey, it beats this next tip we found from one of the nail polish companies from which is…
5. Wear gloves (now there's a practical idea!)
6. Stop wearing polish and wait for your nails to grow out. (Also not too practical, this could take 4 to 6 months.)
7. Soak your nails in 1/2 cup of water and juice of one lemon for up to 15 minutes, once a week, according to Sally Hanson. (We're skeptical if this works but you can always add some sugar and just drink it as lemonade.)
8. Buy only yellow shades of polish so you can't tell if your nails are stained or not. (Sorry, just kidding on that one.)

The Beauty Brains bottom line

Nail polish can stain your nails yellow but by choosing the right shades, using a protective base coat, and drinking a lot of lemonade while wearing gloves, you should be able to control the problem.

Why Did My Nail Polish Remover Stop Working?

Island Girl Wants to Know:
What happened to my polish remover? I use Cutex and now it takes forever to get the polish off.

The Right Beauty Brain Replies:
Our guess is that you might have accidentally bought the wrong Cutex!

Basically, there are two different kinds of nail polish removers: Acetone and Non-Acetone. They work by dissolving the hard film that's left on your nails by the ingredients in the polish.

Acetone
Acetone is a very powerful solvent and it's hands down the best at removing polish. But, it's also very harsh because it removes a lot of natural oils from your skin. In fact, sometimes your skin will look really white if you've used too much acetone on it. That means you've dried it out.

Non-acetone
Non-acetone removers use less aggressive solvents, like ethyl acetate and isopropyl alcohol. They also add moisturizing agents to over come the drying effect. However, these formulations don't dissolve the polish coating as efficiently so you'll have to work harder to take off all the old color.

The Beauty Brains bottom line
To please all consumers, many nail polish remover brands, like Cutex, make both kinds of products. Just be careful to read the label so you know which one you're getting! If you prefer a powerful polish remover look for acetone on the ingredient list and stay away from products that are non-acetone or acetone free.

Chapter 8
Fragrance

What Makes Some Perfumes Last So Long

Jansen Needs Justification:

Hi to both Left and Right Brains, I am currently using a eau de parfum called Allure Homme Sport by Chanel, and it is the MOST long-lasting fragrance ever. (And Yes, I am a bloke). One of my chemist friends told me that this is to do with the exclusive alcohol that Chanel uses in their perfumes, as it probably has a low boiling point and so the fragrances are more volatile. I wonder how true this statement is? Thanks in advanced!

The Left Brain is Left Justified:

Thanks for the question Jansen, it's always a special treat when we hear from our male readers! But while we chemists usually stick together, we have to disagree with your friend's assessment of why Allure lasts so long. To explain why, we have to give you a quick lesson on fragrance chemistry.

Fragrance are complex mixtures of natural and synthetic chemicals designed to create a specific scent. The fragrance ingredients are mixed with alcohol (specifically ethanol) to dilute them to a usable level. Ethanol is used because its safe, it's a good solvent and it evaporates quickly. In fact, the alcohol is the FIRST thing that evaporates. That's why when you first spray on perfume you want to wait a few seconds before smelling it. Otherwise you get a nose full of sharp alcohol odor. As the alcohol flashes off, the other ingredients in the fragrance are more noticeable; these ingredients are loosely grouped into 3 categories depending on how fast they evaporate.

Three notes

Top notes evaporate quickly so you smell them first. These tend to be lighter in nature - think citrus type scents. They are also the first notes to wear out over the course of the day.

Middle notes evaporate a bit slower and create the body of the fragrance, these are usually a combination of floral and/or fruity notes.

Bottom notes are the heavier longer lasting fragrance components. Perfumers describe these notes with terms like woody, balsamic, smoky, or musky. These notes are the "anchors" that help the fragrance last longer. Bingo!

The Beauty Brains bottom line

Allure lasts longer because of the bottom notes in the fragrance not because of the alcohol. And speaking of alcohol, tell your chemist friend he or she should buy you a cocktail to make up for the bad advice!

Feeling Tired? It Might Be What You Smell

Here's a bit of odor research showing that symptoms like fatigue, chest pain and lower back pain may actually be related to the odors you're smelling.

Researchers had 194 people keep track of their stress levels and odor experiences over the course of 8 days. What they found was that physical symptoms actually got worse after people experienced intense odors. They don't know exactly how the two are related but they believe that the memory of the odor becomes linked to the pain which triggers the sensation.

So what can the Beauty Brains community do about it? Well, you might keep a diary like the people in this study did. Anytime you feel fatigued or pain write down all the things that you smell. You may start to notice a pattern and start avoiding odors that trigger the symptoms.

How important is fragrance in your life?

Did you know that about 400,000 people in the US were born without a sense of smell? These people have a condition known as anosmia and effects not only their sense of smell but also their ability to taste. (Here's one author's experience with anosmia). Why most can't smell is mystery but that may be changing.

You can imagine how unfortunate it is, especially when it comes to using perfumes or heavily scented beauty products from places like Lush or Bath & Body Works. Without fragrance people would have a very difficult time noticing any difference between various products.

Does fragrance make the beauty product?
In fact, brands like Philosophy are all about fragrance. Let's compare a couple of their products.

Philosophy Vanilla Birthday Cake 3-in-1 shampoo

Water (aqua), TEA Lauryl Sulfate, PPG 2 Hydroxyethyl Cocamide, Cocamidopropyl Betaine, Glycol Stearate, Disodium Laureth Sulfosuccinate, Sodium Chloride, Glycerin, Glyceryl Polymethacrylate, Fragrance (Parfum), Polyquaternium 7, PEG 150 Distearate, Tocopheryl Acetate, Citric Acid, Sodium Benzotriazolyl Butylphenol Sulfonate, Buteth 3, Tributyl Citrate, Methylchloroisothiazolinone, Methylisothiazolinone, Propylene Glycol, Yellow 5 (CI 19140), Red 40 (CI 16035)

Philosophy Double Rich Hot Cocoa 3-in-1 shampoo

Water (Aqua), TEA Lauryl Sulfate, PPG 2 Hydroxethyl Cocamide, Cocamidopropyl Betaine, Glycol Stearate, Caramel, Disodium Laureth Sulfocsuccinate, Sodium Chloride, Glycerin, Glyceryl Polymethacrylate, Fragrance (Parfum), Polyquaternium 7, PEG 150 Distearate, Tocopheryl Acetate, Citric Acid, Sodium Benzotriazolyl Butylphenol Sulfonate, Buteth 3, Tributyl Citrate, Propylene Glycol, Benzyl Benzoate, Methylchloroisothiazolinone, Methylisothiazolinone, Red 33 (CI 17200)

Notice anything? The formulas are identical except for the color and fragrance. Now, for a non-anosmiatic like myself this is not a problem. I love both of these products. The intense fragrances transport me to happy times; a birthday party when I was 7, a cold winter evening snuggled up by a fire. Oh, such memories from simple body washes.

While anosmiacs won't be able to tell any difference between these two products (except for color), relief may be on the way. Researchers at the Washington DC Taste and Smell Clinic report that they have identified cell death factors in the mucous of anosmiacs. And now they can get to work on finding ways to reduce the effect of these factors.

So if you happen to lose your sense of smell or were unfortunate enough to be born without it, you may be able to take a pill or nasal spray that will allow you to to know the difference between Vanilla Cake and Hot Cocoa shampoo.

Time Travel For Your Nose

Archeologists have discovered a Sephora store from 2000 B.C.

Ok, it's not really Sephora, but it is believed to be the world's oldest perfume factory.

Appropriately located on Cyprus, said to be home to Venus the Goddess of love, this factory still contains the original distilling equipment along with ingredients like olive oil, pine, coriander, laurel, bergamot, parsley and bitter almonds. The laboratory they uncovered is over 40,000 square feet and includes rooms dedicated to olive pressing, copper refining, and fragrance oil storage. According to the researchers, the plant employed dozens of people.

But the really cool thing is that these scientists have used the remnants of this ancient factory to recreate scents that are 4,000 years old. They duplicated the original perfumes using fragrance ingredients extracted from traces left in containers at the site. They even replicated the ancient extraction techniques by steeping the spices in water and oil.

Imagine smelling a fragrance that was made 4000 years ago this may be the closet you'll ever get to actual time travel!

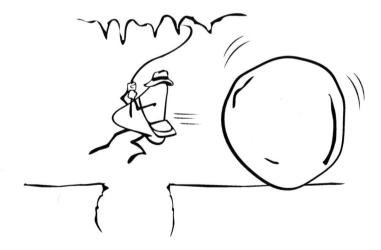

Science and St. Valentines Day - When Chemicals Attract

Could a chemical actually improve your sex life? Well, if a study from San Francisco State University researchers is to be believed it can. According to their work, men are more attracted to women wearing pheromones resulting in more dates, kisses, cuddles and even sex.

What are pheromones

Pheromones are a type of compound that allows animals to chemically communicate with each other. They are versatile chemicals that help ants figure out how to get home, that let dogs mark their territory and that let mammals know when to mate. The word pheromone comes from the Greek words pherin, to transfer, and hormon, to excite. These chemicals are similar to hormones but instead of working within the body, they work between bodies.

How do pheromones work?

The chemical communication of pheromones is simple. One animal (or human) releases the pheromone and another senses it. In essence, the behavior of the sensing animal is controlled by the pheromone releaser. In mammals, pheromones are detected by an organ called vomeronasal organ (VMO) which is located somewhere in the head between the nose and mouth. Pheromones are a bit like odor molecules but they have a much different effect.

So do pheromones really work?

Well, if pheromones really worked it would mean that controlling the behavior of people would be simple. If you wanted someone to fall in love with you, you could simply spray some pheromones whenever they're around. Fortunately, human behavior is a bit more complicated than that.

It is still debated among scientists whether pheromones have an effect or not. These researchers demonstrated that women actually saw an increase in sociosexual activity when wearing perfume that contained pheromones. The impressive part of this research was that it was compared to a placebo control. But one study (of 36 women) isn't enough to substantiate these incredible claims.

Other researchers have looked at all the human pheromone data and the results are inconclusive. Yes, pheromones are real. Yes, they have some physiological effect (such as synchronizing women's menstrual cycles). But how much pheromones change behavior is still unclear.

If it weren't Valentine's Day, I'd be more skeptical on this one, but it is and I really want to believe!

You can search the internet and find lots of sources for pheromone containing products. We're not saying these products will work. In fact, most companies selling pheromones probably don't use real human pheromones anyway. Still, this might just be the thing that helps make this a Valentine's Day to remember.

Science and St. Valentines Day - Living Flowers

Call us corny, but The Beauty Brains still think flowers are a classic Valentines Day gift. Perfume is wonderful, but nothing smells quite as nice as a fresh cut flower. Or does it? Is it possible that modern science can make a perfume that smells just like a real flower?

The answer is yes! Scientists at International Flavors and Fragrance (IFF) one of the world's largest fragrance companies, have developed a new technology that allows them to reproduce the EXACT sent of a living flower - without even having to pick it.

Love and The Living Flower
Floral fragrance ingredients were originally created by picking a flower and processing it to extract the chemical components responsible for its aroma.

While this process did isolate some of the chemicals responsible for the flower's smell, it did not capture the EXACT same scent molecules that were released by the flower and picked up by your nose. That's because a living flower releases different chemicals than a dead, cut flower. Therefore, it was really impossible to replicate the exact scent of fresh flowers.

But IFF's new Living Flower head-space analysis technology changes all that. No, head-space analysis does not refer to some kind of psychoanalytical technique. It's a way of collecting the scent of a living, growing flower instead of just extracting chemicals from a dead flower. It works like this, a large glass globe is placed around the living flower to capture the scent it releases. This globe is connected to a sophisticated Gas Chromatograph that analyzes the exact composition of the scent.

Chemists then use this analysis as a road map to create a synthetic chemical that smells exactly like the original. (This same technique can be applied to fruits as well as flowers.) So instead of chopping up dead flowers, scientists can now create more natural smelling perfumes from living plants. (Hmmm, we wonder if natural perfumes like Le Bijou, Jimmyjane, and Apothena use this technology.) It's another great example of better living (and loving!) through chemistry.

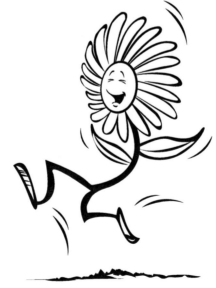

Special fragrance makes you look 12 pounds lighter

One interesting fragrance study suggests that exercise might not be the easiest way to look like you've lost those extra holiday pounds. Dr. Allen Hirsch and his team at the Smell and Taste Treatment and Research foundation have recently found that the perception of body weight could be affect by the fragrance you wear.

In the study, four groups of about 50 men each looked at a woman (actual stats 5'9", 245 lbs) and estimated how much she weighed. With three of the groups the woman was wearing one of three different fragrances (citrus floral, sweet pea/lily of the valley, and floral/spicy). For the fourth group the woman wore no fragrance.

The researchers then compared the weight estimates of each group for differences.

Surprisingly, when the woman wore the floral/spicy fragrance, the men estimated her weight to be 4 pounds less than her actual weight. And if the guys liked the fragrance, they said she looked a full 12 pounds less! Without a single sit-up being done.

Now, this research seems a little weak for my science-minded beauty brain but if repeatable, it is certainly interesting. And even if the results can't be duplicated, it certainly couldn't hurt to start wearing a floral & spice fragrance. I mean, who wouldn't want to spray on a fragrance and look like they lost some weight?

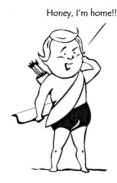

Honey, I'm home!!

Science And St. Valentines Day - Cupid, Cosmetics and Aromatherapy

Everyone knows that Cupid flew around shooting arrows and making people fall in love. But did you also know that Cupid's wife had to sneak into the Underworld and steal cosmetics?

The Myth of Cupid and Cosmetics

It's true, at least according the myth of Cupid and Psyche. It turns out that Cupid's estranged spouse had to travel to Hade's realm and return with Persephone's make up box. Unfortunately, curiosity got the better of her and she couldn't resist opening the forbidden box to see what Persephone kept inside. (Rumor has it that Persephone was fond of Loose Lips lip gloss and Hydroderm Wrinkle Reducer.)

Anyway, Psyche thought if she used some of Persephone's magical makeup, she could win back her husband (hey, she just escaped from Hell, cut her some slack!). Of course, there's always a catch to these myths and when Psyche opened the cosmetic box she was put into a trance and fell into a deep sleep.

The story doesn't end there, fortunately for Cupid. Eventually Psyche eventually woke up and they lived happily ever after. While it's nice to see true love triumph, the myth does leave a nagging question for us science types can cosmetics really relax you enough to make you fall asleep? Believe it or not, modern science suggests that this may actually be possible.

Does Aromatherapy Really Work

According to an article in the April 2004 Issue Of Natural Health, Namni Goel, Ph.D., an assistant professor of psychology and neuroscience at Wesleyan University in Middletown, Conn. conducted a study that indicates that smelling lavender oil can make you sleep more deeply.

His study involved 15 women and 10 men who were asked to intermittently sniff one of two vials for 30 minutes before sleep. One vial contained lavender oil, the other contained an odorless control (the panelists were told this might be a scent diluted so much that it was undetectable.) Then, using electrodes, Goel measured the sleeping panelist's brain waves.

His results showed that the panelists who sniffed lavender oil had significantly increased slow-wave sleep brain patterns which is indicative of a very deep stage of sleep. While this research doesn't mean that lavender can replace sleeping pills, it does indicate there may be a valid scientific basis for some aromatherapy claims.

Chapter 9
Scandals and Secrets of the Beauty Biz

The 3 Biggest Lies That Cosmetic Companies Tell You

Kris' Question:
I'm testing out Arbonne right now, but am thinking I can't afford it. My mother-in-law is a "beauty consultant" for BeautiControl and they seem to have a pretty extensive line of skin care products. Do you know anything about the quality of their line (I'm looking mainly at cleansers, toners, anti-aging products and moisturizers) and/or can you recommend any of their products?

The Left Brain Lashes Out:
Based on what I've seen, the Beauticontrol products seem to be of reasonable quality. They're also very pricey, but if you can afford them, that's

your decision.

What bugs me, and the reason that I would not recommend them, is the way the company hypes their products. I understand the need for creative marketing, but when a company makes statements that border on untrue, that disturbs me. I just hate being lied to and I REALLY hate being lied to under the guise of science. To me there's at least 3 tip offs when a company is stretching the truth about their products. Let me give you some examples using Beauticontrol:

1. Claims of Exclusivity

What's the lie?
They tell that "only" their products can give you a certain benefit.

What's the truth?
The truth is, unless they have a patent or a documented trade secret, they're using the same technology as everyone else in the industry.

What's the example?
Beauticontrol says "only BeautiControl offers comprehensive, customized skin care that addresses what your skin needs when it needs it." Based on their product catalog they appear to have typical cleansers, toners, lotions, etc. that are offered by many, many other companies. Why do they say "only" Beauticontrol offers this kind of treatment?

2. Implying Superior Performance without Substantiation

What's the lie?
They tell you their product works better than anyone else's.

What's the truth?
If they make claims like that they'd better have some kind of proof.

What's the example?

Beauticontrol says "Far beyond traditional dry, combination and oily skin care, BeautiControl takes an innovative, personal approach, to provide total skin wellness through" Blah, blah blah. Again, with conventional products there is no way they can convince me that their products are far beyond traditional ones. Yes, they may be applying a different marketing spin, but there is no technology muscle behind their mouth.

3. "Magic" Ingredient Claims

What's the lie?

They say that some sexy sounding ingredient makes the product work.

What's the truth?

In reality, most of the time it's the formula as a whole and not any single ingredient that makes the product work.

What's the example?

Beauticontrol says one of their products is "formulated with the rejuvenating minerals of the Dead Sea." Minerals don't rejuvenate skin, moisturizing agents do.

Ok, now that I've gotten that out of my system, maybe Beauticontrol isn't "lying" to us (I'm going to catch hell from the Right Brain for this) but they certainly are overstating the uniqueness of their line. And as a scientist, that kind of hype turns me off.

Are You Confused By Organic Products Too?

For chemists like the Beauty Brains, the meaning of 'organic' is clear. It is any chemical compound that contains Carbon. In fact, to get a college chemistry degree you take a year of Organic Chemistry where you memorize endless chemical reactions between hydrocarbons, oxygen, nitrogen and more.

Many a chemist wannabe switched to marketing degrees after flunking organic chemistry.

What does organic mean for cosmetics?

But 'organic' doesn't quite mean the same thing in the cosmetic industry. To consumers it can mean 'natural', 'green', 'chemical free', or 'found at Whole Foods'. But according to this article, the US organics market is completely confused. Primarily because there is no industry-agreed meaning for terms like 'organic' or 'natural'. Unlike the farming industry, these terms are not regulated for cosmetics. Companies can pretty much claim anything is natural or organic.

For example, imagine a body wash formula. It contains all kinds of synthetic surfactants, fragrances, preservatives and colors. But it also contains 85-90% water. A company might simply claim "90% organic or natural" and be telling the truth. Certainly, this isn't in the spirit of what people believe organic to mean, but it is within the law.

Our good friends at Burt's Bees are outraged by the tricks some companies are playing on the public. They are campaigning to get tighter regulations on cosmetics that use terms such as 'natural' or 'organic'. Stay tuned to see if they will make a difference.

Are organic products better?

Incidentally, natural or organic cosmetic products don't really provide any added benefit for consumers. Most companies are just fooling you when they say their products are natural. What isn't? And for companies like Burt's Bees who strive to make 'organic' or 'all-natural' products, their finished products are mostly functionally inferior to more mainstream products. This is the real trade-off of natural or organic products. That and an incredibly higher cost for an inferior product.

Remember cosmetics are not food. No one has ever proven there is a benefit to 'organically' derived cosmetics.

How Beauty Brands Control Your Brain

We frequently field questions asking if expensive name brands are better than other products (See e.l.f. as an example.). Our answers usually deal with the functional aspects of the formulas and we routinely find that there are good and bad quality products at all price points.

Why advertising works

But here's a scientific study we found that sheds some light on WHY people tend to like these expensive (and usually well advertised) brands better. According to this article on brains and branding, researchers at University Hospital in Munich Germany used Magnetic Resonance Imaging technology to scan people's brains while they were shown different brand logos. The more popular logos "lit up areas of the brain associated with warm emotions, reward and self-identity while less-recognized brands triggered more activity in brain regions associated with working memory and negative emotions — suggesting these products were less easy to process and accept. Hmmm. Maybe that explains why I start to drool when looking at the Tiffany catalog.

The Beauty Brains bottom line

This study is part of a new scientific trend called neuroeconomics in which psychologists, neuroscientists, radiologists and marketing experts work together to unravel the mysteries of the consumer's mind. Fascinating stuff but just a little bit scary!

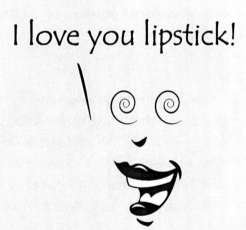

I love you lipstick!

5 Home Beauty Gadgets That Really Work

Megan's Musing:
I've read that an at-home tool called a Wellbox is supposed to help reduce the appearance of cellulite. Has anyone tried this device with promising results, or is this a waste of (significant) money?

The Right Brain Responds:
Megan, we've blogged about cellulite treatments before, and they really don't do much. At best they only give you a very minor, temporary effect so you should probably save your money. But you might be interested to know that there ARE several new beauty gadgets on the market that really do work. At least according to a Dermatology Times article that quotes Dr. Thomas Rohrer, M.D., clinical associate professor of dermatology, Boston University Medical Center. He says that "We are getting to the point where, for certain things, patients may be able to treat themselves safely and fairly effectively at home."

However, Dr. Rohrer also points out that these treatments are still less effective than the devices used by physicians: "They're not going to be nearly as powerful" but "they may be effective enough…to improve some conditions." Here are 5 beauty gadgets that Dr. Rohrer says really work:

1. Hair-removal (the Epila SI 808 Laser and the Spa Touch from Radiancy)
According to Dr. Rohrer, Spa Touch showed moderate efficacy with patients reporting an average 66% reduction in unwanted hair counts. At nine months follow-up, patients noted about a one-third reduction. Furthermore, there were a minimal side effects.

2. Hair loss (HairMax LaserComb from Lexington International LLC)
This device is one of only three treatments that are FDA-approved for hair growth. Dr. Rohrer says that "in a 26-week, multi-center, placebo-controlled study with this device, 93 percent of subjects noticed an increase in hair count."

3. Acne devices (Zeno from Tyrell and ClearTouch Lite from Radiancy)
Both devices thermally treat acne lesions and according to the Dr., Zeno achieved 90 percent reduction in lesion counts in one to two days.

4. Facial photo-rejuvenation (NuLase from NuLase International LLC and ClearTouch Lite from Radiance) Light Emitting Diode devices are safe, relatively pain-free, and can provide "subtle but real changes in the skin."

5. Facial Toning (Facial Toning Device from Radiancy) Dr. Rohrer claims the Radiancy devices uses LHE technology and is capable of reducing age spots and wrinkles. However, the study he cited has not yet been published so we're more skeptical on this one.

How Salon Brands Get Away With Lying To You

A comment from a salon operator who's concerned about L'Oreal buying Pureology:
I just noticed that the first ingredient listed in the Pureology shampoos and conditioners is now water. It`s crazy how L'Oreal buys them and the first thing they do is "water down" the product (but not the price). My clients loved that there was no water in the products because they so concentrated. They really liked the first ingredient listed being certified botanical extracts. I guess I'll have to switch my Pureology clients over to something else because it's no longer unique.

The Left Brain responds:
I certainly can't tell you what products you should recommend for your clients, but as a scientist I do want to help you understand the science of what you're selling.

Small companies can be sneaky
The old Pureology shampoos and conditioners are good, although over-priced, products. But just because the first ingredient is a botanical blend

instead of water doesn't mean the products are more concentrated. And it certainly doesn't mean the products didn't contain any water!

What it really means is that Pureology was a small independent salon company, and they chose not to strictly follow the cosmetic labeling laws. Many small companies use this trick of listing extracts first, thus making it look like they don't have any water. Don't fall for it! It's one of the oldest tricks in this industry and it's misleading and unfair. The formula is still mostly water!

Unfortunately, the Federal Trade Commission (FTC) and other agencies that fight this kind of consumer fraud are too busy with more serious issues and don't have time to chase after small companies who are tricking consumers with these kind of labeling lies.

Bigger companies follow the law

Since L'Oreal is a much bigger company they tend to play by the rules that all the big companies are held to. In the end, this is better for the consumer because you're getting more truth. Instead of being upset with L'Oreal, you should be thankful that they're labeling the products honestly.

And by the way, since L'Oreal has a much larger research staff than Pureology, any formula changes they made are probably for the better!

The Beauty Brains bottom line

As we've said many times, if you like a product and you can afford it, buy it. But if you're buying a product because of hype you hear from the company that sells it, you're being fooled. Save your money and buy something less expensive!

7 Ways To Hack Your Broken Beauty Products

Our friends at Real Simple magazine have a great online series about how to fix broken beauty products. They describes the cause of each problem, how to fix it, and how to take steps to prevent it from happening again. Nicely done, Real Simple!

Here is the list along with a few comments of our own. You can go to the Real Simple webpage to see their summary and pictures.

1. Broken Lipstick
After you make the repairs they suggest, you can make your lipstick shine like new by VERY CAREFULLY passing it over a candle flame. Kids don't try this at home!

2. Clogged Hairspray Pump
In addition to what Real Simple says, you should also know that a clogged hairspray can also be caused by a poorly designed formula. The resin that holds your hair in place can separate out if it's not properly neutralized. If this is the case you'll see little white specks floating in the product. Throw it away, it can't be fixed!

3. Jammed Lotion Pump
Of course you can also switch a pump from another skin lotion product.

4. Broken Perfume Pump
They didn't mention that the heat can cause the diptube (the thin plastic straw that carries the product up to the pump) to swell up and become sealed shut. Store perfume in a cool place.

5. Shattered Powder Eye Shadow or Blush
If you're following their tip and you apply alcohol to the eye shadow compact, make sure you let it dry completely. Alcohol might carry in enough water to let bacteria grow in the powder cake.

6. Missing or Broken Aerosol Cap
They say aerosol "cap" but they're really talking about the button or the actuator, as it is technically known. The cap is the piece that covers the entire top of the can.

7. Stuck Nail-Polish Lid
We agree with their comments. You might also try rubbing a little nail polish remover under the edge of the lid before trying to loosen it. You won't get much under there, but it might help.

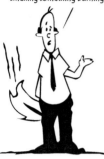

Am I the only one smelling something burning?!!

Garnier Nutritioniste: Liar, Liar Pants On Fire?

SJP wants to know:

I love it when you tell us the real scoop on advertising so I'm curious what you think about Garnier Nutritioniste Ultra-Lift. Their advertising says "It's skin care that actually lifts wrinkles from the inside out." How can they say this?

The Left Brain replies:

They can't say it, at least not anymore. According to the August 20, 2007 edition of the Rose Sheet (a cosmetic industry bulletin) L'Oreal has been asked to modify or discontinue certain claims for Nutritioniste Ultra lift and Skin Renew products by the NAD (National Advertising Division). Here's a quick recap of the issues with 3 of L'Oreal's claims:

1. "…it actually lifts wrinkles from the inside out"
What the NAD says: *"It is well established that topical creams do not absorb deep inside the skin in the same manner as cosmetic fillers such as collagen injections."* In other words, this lotion works from the outside in, not the other way around!

2. "…in three weeks wrinkles are visibly lifted and skin is noticeably firmer"
What the NAD says: *In L'Oreal's clinical study the questions "related to skin firmness refer to skin feeling firmer, not being noticeably firmer as is explicitly stated in one of the challenged claims."*

3. Ultra lift "refuels cells within skin's deepest surface layers"
What the NAD says: *L'Oreal's 9 week study showed Ultra Lift's effect on fine line, shallow wrinkles, and tactile roughness, and skin laxity. This is inadequate "particularly with regard to hydration - despite the presence of moisture locking ingredients Omega 3 and 6."*

To be fair, I should point out that the NAD is not saying this product doesn't work at all. For example, they did recognize that "scientific articles presented by the advertiser provide a reasonable basis for it's ingredient claims in terms of accelerated cell proliferation and upped collagen production." It's just that L'Oreal didn't have adequate support for all the claims that they were making and so they have been asked to change their advertising.

5 Fascinating Facts About Max Factor Cosmetics

Connie wants to win:
Can you please settle a bet? My friend is trying to convince me that the Max Factor cosmetic line is really named after a guy named Max Factor. Sounds like an urban legend to me. I'm guessing it's really a marketing name like "Maximum Coverage Factor" or something like that. Please answer quickly, I can win an Itunes gift card!

The Left Brain resolves the bet:
You can also LOSE an iTunes gift card, Connie. I'm afraid your friend is right: Max Factor Cosmetics is actually named after the chemist who created it: Max Faktor.

Max is actually quite famous among us cosmetic chemists as one of the early pioneers of modern makeup. Here are few fun historical facts:

Faktor to Factor
Born in Poland in 1877, by the age of 20 Max was selling handmade rouges, fragrances and wigs. He came to the US in 1902 where he changed his name from "Faktor" to "Factor" and by 1904 he was selling lotions and hair care products at the St. Louis World's Fair.

Shoot for the stars
In 1914 he created the first line of grease paint products designed for motion picture stars. In just a few short decades, Jean Harlow, Claudette

Colbert, Bette Davis, and virtually all of the major movie actresses were regular customers of the Max Factor beauty salon, located near Hollywood Boulevard.

He made up make up
In the 1920s he developed a new line of color cosmetics for use in the new field of color motion pictures. In fact, he is credited with coining the word "makeup."

Max and Oscar
In 1928 he was awarded a special technology Oscar from the Academy of Motion Picture Arts and Sciences for his make up inventions. (Imagine that – a cosmetic chemist winning an Academy Award!)

Selling like hotcakes
In the 1930's he developed the first powder makeup in solid form, also known as Pancake Makeup, for film stars. When he made it available to the general public, Pancake Makeup became of the biggest selling products in the history of the cosmetic industry. - *Sorry about the iTunes card!*

Are Arbonne products the best skin care you can buy?

Wenditha wonders:
Hey Left! Thanks for telling me about The Beauty Brains site. It's great! Very pretty too, what with all the pink. :) So I'm wondering about a beauty company called Arbonne? Could you tell me what the Beauty Brains think? They're supposed to be the end-all, be-all, but I remain cautious. However, I've used some samples of their anti-aging skin line and found it to be very nice.

Left Beauty Brain responds:
Thanks for the question. We looked into the Arbonne products and have this to say.

The Arbonne Company

First, Arbonne is one of these multi-level marketing companies like Amway in which you are encouraged to become a salesperson, have parties and recruit other people to become salespeople. I've always been skeptical of these kinds of schemes but here's a guy who has an interesting perspective on Arbonne on becoming an Arbonne salesperson. Personally, I wonder why the products aren't sold in the normal way through department or grocery stores. This would certainly make it easy to ignore the truth in advertising rules that other companies who sell through stores need to follow.

The Arbonne Marketing Story

Based on the information on their website, Arbonne products are claimed to be premium skin care products are formulated in Switzerland at the Arbonne Institute of Research and Development (AIRD) and made in the U.S.A.

They follow the standard all-natural marketing story that you find from every other natural company, although they imply some kind of advanced science as if there was any. All the usual claims about how great their products are here. We've previously discussed cosmetic claims and what they really mean.

Here is a sampling of their claims.
1. Botanically based: based on botanical and herbal principles. This doesn't really mean anything. What are botanical & herbal principles?
2. pH correct. Big deal. So is every other skin care product.
3. Dermatologist tested. Just like everyone else's product.
4. Formulated without dyes, animal products, fragrances, mineral oil. Again, more stuff that everyone else says.

The thing that's different about these products than a mass market brand like Aveeno is the price. Arbonne is a whopping $19.50 for 8 ounces! Aveeno is $9.99 for 18 ounces. Functionally, there will likely be no noticeable difference.

The Arbonne Products

The problem with these products is that they don`t live up to their natural claims. While we here at The Beauty Brains think stories about the trouble with chemicals like SLS and parabens are overblown, the natural crowd does not feel similarly. Arbonne formulas fail in this regard because they contain all kinds of chemicals that those people are afraid of. This review of Arbonne products spells it all out from their perspective. Of course, this fact has no bearing on whether the products are good or not, but it certainly suggests their marketing is suspect.

So, what about the products? Are they worth the extra money? Scientifically speaking, they're probably not.

It was difficult to find the ingredient lists because they are not on their main website. However, here is one we found related to their skin lotion.

Arbonne Skin Moisturizing Lotion

Ingredients: *Water, Carthamus Tinctorius (Safflower) Seed Oil, Glyceryl Stearate, PEG-100 Stearate, Aloe Barbadensis Leaf Juice, Cetearyl Alcohol, Ceteareth-20, Glycerin, Butyrospermum Parkii (Shea Butter) Fruit, Althaea Officinalis Root Extract, Chamomilla Recutita (Matricaria) Extract, Taraxacum Officinale (Dandelion) Extract, Glycyrrhiza Glabra (Licorice) Extract, Rosmarinus Officinalis (Rosemary) Leaf Extract, Salvia Officinalis (Sage) Leaf Extract, Retinyl Palmitate, Ergocalciferol, Tocopheryl Acetate, Panthenol, Prunus Amygdalus Dulcis (Sweet Almond) Oil, Olea Europaea (Olive) Fruit Oil, Zea Mays (Corn) Oil, Persea Gratissima (Avocado) Oil, Rosa Damascena Flower Oil, Stearic Acid, Cetyl Alcohol, Ethylhexyl Salicylate, Polysorbate 60, Carbomer, Disodium EDTA, Dimethicone, Quaternium-15, Triethanolamine*

This is a standard lotion complete with water, fatty alcohols, oils, emulsifiers, thickeners and preservatives. All of the natural sounding ingredients are most likely in there at such low levels they don't really do anything. And even if they were in there at higher levels there is no proof that they would have a ny special effect anyway.

The Beauty Brains bottom line
Arbonne is not the end-all be all of skin care or any other personal care product. They are good formulas, but pretty standard and will not perform noticeably better than the products you can buy at your local grocery store. Buy them if you like (they'll work fine) but don't kid yourself into thinking they are anything special, they're not. And if you're looking to start your own business, forget multi-level marketing schemes. Check out the excellent website Start Up Nation instead.

Does Technology Make Arbonne Products Different?

There are certain topics on the Beauty Brains that spark vigorous debate. Supporters provide a tenacious defense of their favorite products despite limited proof of effectiveness. Jan Marini and the eyelash growth product is one and Arbonne products are another. This post concerns the later.

Recently, we received an email from Christine who is a self-proclaimed Arbonne representative. She is proud to report that she's a true believer who has "drunk the Koolaid". You can see all of her comments in our previous Arbonne post.

She took issue with the fact that we suggested Arbonne products really weren't much different than store brands. We'd like to respond to some points made in her comments because they are instructive in how to be a skeptical cosmetic consumer.

What does it mean to research a topic?
I spent three years of law school learning how to learn, so I researched Arbonne quite thoroughly before deciding to jump in with both feet

We hear this claim fairly often. People write in and explain how they've researched a product. Unfortunately, they rarely describe what was involved in this research. Did they go to the website and just read what was published by the marketing department of the company? Did they go to internet forums and see what people were posting about the products? Did they just read opinions on beauty blogs or hear something from their stylist? While these sources are helpful for product information, they are not really "research". Each of these is full of biased opinions that may or may not be reliable.

Real research is a combination of product information plus intimate knowledge of raw materials, familiarity with formulating techniques, and experience with numerous laboratory evaluation techniques. Ideally, there would even be peer reviewed research published in a journal like those found at PubMed.

Here at the Beauty Brains we try to use our background in product formulation and sometimes even actual laboratory product evaluations to generate our opinions. Christine is correct to say that these are still just "subjective opinions" but unlike most, we have no products to sell you and we are not trying to convince ourselves we didn't overpay for a product. Hopefully, this allows us to provide the most unbiased evaluations possible.

Is the technology really different?
The commenter makes the point that there are "THREE KEY THINGS" that make Arbonne different. Only one of these has to do with the product.

The first thing is Arbonne's technology, and the delivery system of the product. Most beauty products are made up of great ingredients - they can be the best on the market. However, they often do not penetrate directly to the epidermal cells that need the moisture the most. The do not self-adjust. Arbonne uses a technology called Nanosphere technology - look it up... The nanosphere technology takes the medication, or the product, in our case, directly to the cellular areas that need it the most. Arbonne's moisturizers do not sit on the skin like most other brands do. The product not only penetrates down from the top epidermal level, but does its work where it is needed the most. Superior product? Not necessarily.

Superior delivery? Definitely.

It's common for people to tell us that their technology is different. Arbonne's "superior" technology is a thing they call Nanospheres. But this is the same type of technology that companies like L'Oreal and P&G have. This doesn't make them different.

And while nanosphere technology may sound superior to some, it scares many experts in the nanotechnology field. In the US, nanotechnology is unregulated even though it has the potential to cause unexpected harm. You don't want your cosmetics to penetrate your skin! When they do, they can get into your body and potentially cause harm. Superior technology does not penetrate. At present, we recommend you avoid products that say they contain nanotechnology.

Finally, despite the safety concerns of nanotechnology there is still no proof that Arbonne moisturizers, body washes or shampoos work any better than typical store brands. Could someone show us an independent side-by-side study comparing Arbonne moisturizers to Olay?

The Beauty Brains bottom line:
There is no doubt that Arbonne produces a high quality product. However, we stand behind our original assessment that they are technologically not much different than brands you can get at the store. With the exception of sunscreen, we also suggest you avoid cosmetics that claim to have nanotechnology.

Chapter 10
Cosmetic Surgery

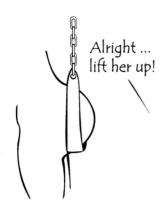

Alright ...
lift her up!

Buy Better Buttocks
With A Brazilian Butt Lift

Claire's question:
My sister Grace told me she's considering a plastic surgery procedure to improve her posterior. What can you tell me about the Brazilian Butt Lift?

The Right Brain butts in:
Claire, normally we try to focus on cosmetic products but it's hard to resist an email that combines the terms "Brazilian" and "Butt" in the same question. So, we checked with our favorite cosmetic surgeon, Dr. Tony Youn, for the 411 on butt lifting.

What is a Brazilian Butt Lift?

As the name implies, it's a procedure to shape and firm your derrière. We wonder why it's named after this particular country. Was it first performed by doctors in Brazil? Do Brazilian women have genetically superior asses? Or is the process some how related to Brazil nuts? We can only speculate…

Whatever the derivation of its name, a BBL is designed to give you "youthful, prominent, perky buttocks." How does it work? Fat grafting! That means the surgeon uses liposuction to remove fat from your lower back, stomach and thighs. The fat is purified and then re-injected into different areas of your buttocks at various depths. It may take hundreds of tiny injections to fill the upper quadrant of your buttocks but when done correctly it does make your butt look better. But a poor injection job can be painful and produce fat shapeless buttocks.

Are there any problems with this perky pooper procedure?

Aside from the aforementioned shapeless buttocks, other side effects include irregular asymmetric skin, numbness, bruising and swelling. On occasion, the incisions may ooze significant fluid. And since the doctor may need to overfill your buttocks to allow for some fat re-absorption back into your body, your butt may temporarily look puffy or swollen. The good news is that unlike silicone butt implants, there is no risk of allergic reaction since the fat injections are your own natural substance.

To avoid some of these issues Dr Youn says: "My favorite way to enhance the buttocks, however, is to liposuction the hips and thighs around it. This essentially makes everything around it smaller, and can indirectly make the bottom look bigger and rounder compared to the rest of the body. It doesn't take as much time, has few complications, and allows the patient to sit down immediately."

How many bucks will it cost to lift my butt?

According to what we found on other sites (these are not Dr. Youn's prices), the average cost of a Brazilian Butt Lift is about $15,000. That includes the physician's fee, anesthesia, hospital costs, post operative nursing care, and all post operative office visits.

So tell your sister that for the price of a new car, she can have the rear end of her dreams.

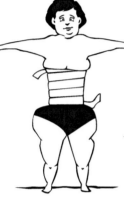

Can Mesotherapy Magically Melt Away Fat?

Deb A. asks:
Do you have much knowledge on a therapy for skin tightening known as Mesotherapy? Apparently they have been doing it for many years in France and recently brought it to the US. It is a series of injections with a drug "cocktail" containing homeopathic and chemicals (including hyaluronic acid) to stimulate skin tightening and collagen production.

The Left Brain trims the fat:
According to The American Society of Plastic Surgeons, Mesotherapy has not been established as safe and effective. I quote:

According to an ASPS Device & Technique Assessment (DATA) Committee report published in the April 15 (2005) issue of Plastic and Reconstructive Surgery patients should be wary of mesotherapy until the safety and effectiveness of the procedure are confirmed.

The following line caught my attention:
There is no information on what happens to fatty acids once they leave the targeted area or how the various ingredients affect the body's organs and other tissues. There is simply too much we do not know about mesotherapy to say it is unquestionably safe for patients.

More recently (August 2006) the American Academy of Dermatologists had this to say Mesotherapy:

Dr. Donofrio notes that a precise definition of the term is lacking "from her perspective it may be considered a subcutaneous injection technique of any medication, in any locale of the body, with the goal of removing fat (cellulite) or having an anti-aging effect... There is very sparse medical literature on the efficacy of mesotherapy.

The article goes on to site examples of mesotherapy injections with different materials gave different kinds of results. At best it sounds like the process is inconsistent, at worse it sounds dangerous.

The conclusion of the article really sums up what I think:

What can we advise our patients who inquire about the potential benefits of mesotherapy? Perhaps sometime in the future, a brilliant innovator will have the developed the proper cocktail that, when injected into the subcutaneous tissue, will cause lipolysis, in a risk-free manner. That day has not arrived. In 2006, regarding mesotherapy, only two words prevail: caveat emptor.

The Beauty Brains bottom line

Perhaps new information has come to light in the last year, but I didn't find it. So, considering the lack of solid medical data on this process, I'd be very careful. There really isn't enough evidence to say that it's worth doing.

The Top 5 Causes Of Droopy Eyelids

Big Evie Is Feeling Droopy:
Aside from surgical procedures, what's the best way to lift eyelids that are just beginning to sag? I notice that my eyelids perk up after a nap, but I can't sleep all of the time!

- continued

The Right Brain Lifts Her Spirits:
A saggy or droopy eyelid is also called ptosis or blepharoptosis. For most people this condition is just annoying but when the it's severe, the lowered lid can actually interfere with your vision. There are 5 primary types of ptosis, each with it's own cause:

1. Congenital ptosis
This affects infants and occurs when the levator muscle (the muscle that lifts the eyelid) doesn't develop properly. Surgery may be required to prevent permanent loss of vision later in the child's life.

2. Muscle diseases
This condition is like myasthenia gravis, progressive external ophthalmoplegia, or oculopharyngeal muscular dystrophy, can cause ptosis too. These conditions are much more serious and ptosis os more of a side effect than the actual problem. Seek medical help if you think you have any muscular disorder. Cosmetic Surgery

3. Nerve problems
These can cause ptosis because the eye muscles are controlled by nerves. Any condition that damages the nerves, like a stroke, brain tumor, brain aneurysm can result in ptosis.

4. Local eye problems
Special conditions like eye infections, tumors inside the eye socket, or even a blow to the eye, can cause ptosis as well.

5. Aponeurotic ptosis
Also called senile or age-related ptosis, aponeurotic ptosis is the most common type. The combination of gravity and aging results in a stretches the tendon-like tissue that helps the levator muscle hold the eyelid open. Hard contact lenses, history of eye infections, of trauma to the eye can increase chances of this type of ptosis.

The Beauty Brains bottom line
Because gravity and old age are such powerful forces, The Beauty Brains think the most likely cause of your problem is the Age-Related type (We hate to call it the Senile Type!) But if your problem is severe, or if you're having any other symptoms, you shouldn't hesitate to see a doctor. Unfortunately, short of having eye surgery there's really no effective treatment for droopy eyelids. Some film forming cosmetics may give you temporary respite by providing a slight tightening of the eyelid skin, but there's no topical product that can truly reverse this condition.

Are Stem Cells Better Than Silicone?

You've probably heard about the problems with saline or silicone implants (rupturing, leaking, interfering with mammograms). And then there is the issue of them not looking natural. Well, researchers at the University of Illinois at Chicago have been investigating the problem and have reportedly come up with a solution. Dr. Jeremy Mao and his team of researchers have discovered that they can create superior implants by using cells from a patient's own body.

The way it works is they remove a few bone marrow stem cells from your body. Then they grow these cells in a bio-scaffolding (which is just a fancy Petri dish). The scaffolding can be molded to any size or shape and over time the cells multiply and grow to that shape. When the implant is ready (after a few weeks) it is put in the body and will work just like natural breast tissue.

Of course the research is in its early stages and more long term studies will have to be completed. But the researchers are close. Someday, really natural new breasts made from your own cells will be a reality.

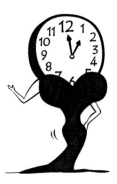

One Hour to Bigger Breasts?

Oh now come on, this just doesn't sound right. I saw this article about a new technology for lunch hour boob jobs and was simultaneously intrigued, disturbed, and skeptical. One hour for bigger breasts? Really?

According to the article a company called Cytori Therapeutics says they have a stem-cell based technology that can actually super-charge your fat cells and fill in breast volume. The way it works is this. First, fat is taken from the patient's butt or stomach via liposuction. Then stem cells from the fat are isolated and put into a small cartridge. This is then injected into the breasts. The whole procedure takes a little over an hour. Then during the next 6 months the stem cells grow and somehow make the breasts get larger. Clinical trials are reportedly under way and the process has already been approved in Germany. This sounds very similar to a breast technology we discussed last year.

Brains are skeptical
The thing that gets my skeptical senses going is that this wasn't published in any of the typical science wires that the Beauty Brains frequent. The story cites Chemistry and Industry magazine as their source. This is a less-scientific source than journals like Science or Nature or The New England Journal of Medicine where you might expect a big story like this to break. Chemistry and Industry Magazine tends to hype technologies without solid science to back it up.

So, I looked into Cytori Therapeutics. They're based in California (of course, the world capital of boob jobs) and they call the technology the Celution System. Med Gadget did a report on the Celution technology last year and said it had not yet been proven to work. But this report from the BBC indicates a 19 person trial conducted in Japan showed it basically worked with no major side effects. That's a small number but encouraging. More testing is needed.

The Beauty Brains bottom line
Interesting and it may actually work. It won't be available for another couple years but can you imagine, new breasts in under an hour with no cutting? How many in the Beauty Brains community would sign up for that?

How Can You Tell if Someone Has Breast Implants?

Suzie M Wants To Know:
This is a little bit embarrassing, but I'd like to know how to tell when someone has had a boob job. My friends think they can spot fake ones a mile away, but I'm not so sure. Are there any technical tip offs that we should know about?

The Right Boob, uh, I mean Brain, Replies:
We're cosmetic scientists, not cosmetic surgeons, but we did some research and we think we can help on this one. A lot of this information is common sense, but we've tried to look at this as scientifically as possible.

First let's point out that factors such as body type, original breast size and shape, and type and placement of the implant are important in the resulting appearance. And of course, don't underestimate the skill and experience of the surgeon. Having said that, there are a few key things to look for when deciding if someone's breasts are Real or Real Expensive.

In the interest of good taste, we'll limit this discussion to observations you can make on a woman who's fully clothed and not talk about how you can tell from touching them or from things you could see on a naked breast, like scars.

1. Size
While size alone can't tell you if breasts have been augmented or not, it certainly is an important factor. Pay attention to whether or not a woman's breasts look disproportionate to her body. If they look too big and you want to know if they're fake, consider the rest of the visual cues listed below.

2. Shape
Is the shape too perfect? If so, they might be fake since the majority of natural breasts aren't perfect orbs. Furthermore, real breasts are not exactly identical, so if they look like perfect twins they might be artificial. Also

look for too much roundness as opposed to a more relaxed pear-like shape. Natural breasts have a natural sliding curve line from top to bottom. They slope down gradually. Implants tend to have a much higher arc as you look from top to bottom. Firm appearance is another cue; augmented breasts can look more like solid muscle.

3. Placement
Vertical placement: Look at where the breast are positioned on her chest. Breasts are naturally found at about armpit height. Frequently, implants are placed too high on the chest. This is particularly noticeable if she's not wearing a bra. Horizontal placement: look at the spacing between the breasts. If they're more than a fist's width apart, they might be fake. If the surgeon didn't properly scrape the pectoral tendons, the implants may not be spaced close enough together.

4. Movement
Real breasts are mostly fat, which gives them a jiggle quality; implants don't move that way. Look at the way her breasts shift (or don't shift) when she she reaches back or stretches. If they maintain the same dimensions, instead of flattening out, then they're probably fake. Observe how they follow her body movements, particularly when she's moving and swinging her arms. Watch how they behave as she bends over, you should see them fall if they're real. If you're looking at someone at who's laying down at the beach or the pool or whatever, see if her breasts naturally fall to the side or if they unnaturally stick up.

5. Other Visual Cues
Depending on what she's wearing, you might be able to see some additional visual cues like the shape and location of her nipples. A bad boob job may put them too high, too low, or not pointing in the same direction. You might also be able to catch a glimpse of stretch marks that could be a byproduct of the surgery. (Of course, stretch marks can also occur naturally from weight gain and loss.)

Take the Quiz

Think you've got it now? Then take this online quiz on Augmentation Mammoplasty (http://www.controlledmedia.com/pages/mammoplastyhtm). You get to guess if 30 different pairs of breasts are natural or augmented. Good luck!

Can Brava Give You Better Boobs?

Andrea asks:
I would like to have a larger bust, but I really don't want implants. I have heard of the Brava Breast Enhancement system, which seems to be endorsed by a lot of plastic surgeons, and some scientific studies. Do you have any inside info or insight?

The Left Brain responds:
If we keep getting questions about bras and breast enhancement I'll have to add a special Boob category on the sidebar!

For those of you in the Beauty Brains community who are not familiar with the Brava system, it supposedly works by gently pulling on your breasts which keeps them under tension for hours at a time. This sustained tension causes the cells to grow new tissue that makes your breasts appear larger and fuller.

How does BRAVA work
According to the the BRAVA website, the System consists of two semi-rigid domes, with specially engineered silicone gel rims, and a sophisticated minicomputer, called a SmartBox, that creates and regulates the tension within the domes.

Semi-rigid domes? Engineered silicone rims? Sophisticated minicomputer? Is this a breast enhancer or some kind of Terminator Robot from the Future?

But I digress. The real question is, does it really work? Since our forte is cosmetic chemistry, not breast enhancement, we asked our friend Dr. Rob Oliver over at Plastic Surgery 101 to give his expert opinion. Based on his experience, Dr. Rob says that Brava doesn't work well, it's uncomfortable, and must be worn for weeks before you see results if you see any at all. He's aware of very few people who use or endorse it.

The Beauty Brains bottom line

That's good enough for me - I'll take the opinion of a doctor and scientist over the hype from the company selling the product any day. Dr. Rob said he'd try to post more details on his blog, so keep your eye on Plastic Surgery 101. If you haven't used it, I suggest you save your money.

Cosmetic Surgery And The Suicide Connection

There was a fascinating New Scientist article about a possible connection between cosmetic surgery and suicide. According to researchers women who get breast implants are 2 to 3 times more likely to commit suicide than woman who don't. This same connection was found in 5 independent studies suggesting there may actually be something to it. There was even a suggestion that this value may be higher because women who have breast implants were also more likely to get into fatal car accidents. These would typically be reported as accidents when they could possibly be suicides.

So it leads to the question, why would there be a connection? The following were proposed as possible reasons.

1. Undiagnosed psychological problems
This was said to be the most likely cause. Women who elect to get cosmetic surgery like this are more likely to have some kind of psychological disorder. This includes a condition called body dysmorphic disorder (BDD) in which a person obsesses about barely noticeable or non-existent flaws in their appearance.

2. Drugs & Alcohol
Women who get breast implants are also more likely to partake in drugs & alcohol. It could be that these are the real culprit and the breast implants are just coincidence.

3. Implant leaks
While the scientists say this is highly unlikely it hasn't been ruled out. It is possible that the chemicals in breast implants are leaking out, affecting the brain, and triggering suicide.

Amazingly, 291,000 American women had breast implants last year. This side of the Beauty Brains has to wonder, Is it really worth it?

Thankfully, there are push-up bras and other non-surgical options to make them look bigger. On the other hand, people should just accept each other for how they are. But be sure to keep using make-up and other cosmetics. You wouldn't want the Beauty Brains to be out of a job right?

Chapter 11
Cosmetic Concerns

Are Your Cosmetics Poisoning You?

"Women absorb up to 5 pounds of damaging chemicals a year from their beauty products."

I saw this newspaper headline and was amazed, astonished, and perplexed. I just couldn't believe it. Being a skeptical Brain, I figured the article was just a typical "scare" piece designed to spook us into fearing chemicals, but they actually provide a reference to their headline and quotes from a biochemist. So, this Beauty Brain was intrigued. Are we really absorbing pounds of chemicals through our skin? I had to see their proof. The actual quote from the article is as follows:

"The average woman absorbs 4lb 6oz of chemicals from toiletries and make-up every year, the industry magazine In-Cosmetics recently reported."

Question the source

Here's where it gets interesting. First of all, In-Cosmetics is not a peer-reviewed scientific journal, it's a magazine published in conjunction with an annual trade show where companies that sell cosmetic ingredients go to show off their newest products. Secondly, the quote appeared in this article "Trends in natural and organic cosmetics and toiletries."

It turns out, the notion that women absorb 5 pounds of chemicals from cosmetics comes from a scientist who runs a natural company called Spiezia Organics. According to Dr. Mariano Spiezia and his wife Loredana "everything we need to be fulfilled and healthy is provided by nature. Today's research suggests that the human body will absorb most of what is applied to the skin, meaning that up to 2kg (5 pounds) of chemicals a year from toiletries and skincare preparations used daily."

There is no other reference provided. No studies are cited. Dr. Spiezia makes this assertion without any data at all. Then the reporter completely believes the statement and quotes it as fact.

It is not fact. It is nonsense. It is the kind of junk science that some Natural or Organic companies try to dupe you with so you won't feel bad about spending your hard earned money on their over-priced products.

Do you absorb 5 lbs of cosmetic chemicals through your skin?

Based on our knowledge of the barrier properties of skin, this claim seems ridiculous. It suggests skin is a sponge that absorbs any chemical it's exposed to. In fact, skin is the opposite. It is actually a barrier that prevents chemicals from getting inside your body.

It's not a perfect barrier because some compounds do pass through the skin like some sunscreens (eg. benzophenone-3) and drugs like Nicotine.

Even caffeine can enter your blood stream through your skin. So scientists are concerned about chemicals on the skin. But safety studies are conducted chemicals all the time and the vast majority don't behave as such.

For the most part, cosmetic raw materials do not penetrate the skin so deep that they are absorbed into the blood stream. They typically absorb into only the top layer of skin (stratum corneum) and are naturally removed over time.

The Beauty Brains bottom line
No, your cosmetics are not poisoning you. While chemicals can absorb into your skin, it is true of only a small number of them and these have not been shown to cause problems. You certainly don't absorb 5 lbs of chemicals through your skin; we'll try to assess how much you really do absorb and report back after a bit more research. But the important thing is when you hear claims like this in the media, be sure to check the source. Occasionally, it's backed up by science, but usually it is propaganda by a biased source. Proof is found in scientific studies not in the opinions of natural-product selling "experts".

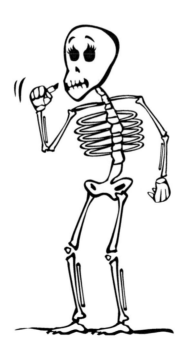

Common Cosmetic Skin Irritants

How many of you Beauty Brains faithful have experienced some kind of temporary skin rash, reddening, or itchiness? That condition is known as allergic contact dermatitis and a recent study by the Mayo Clinic lists the top 10 ingredients that can cause this condition. The list includes metals, antibiotics, fragrance ingredients, and various preservatives. If you experience this condition the best solution is to avoid these ingredients!

Top 10 Skin Irritants

1. Nickel (nickel sulfate hexahydrate): Found in jewelry or on your clothes.

2. Gold (gold sodium thiosulfate): Yes, the same stuff used to make jewelry.

3. Cobalt chloride: A metal used for many applications like medical products, hair dye, and antiperspirants to name a few.

4. Neomycin sulfate: An antibiotic used in various first aid creams. Less commonly used in cosmetics.

5. Bacitracin: Another antibiotic.

6. Thimerosal: An ingredient used in antiseptics and vaccines

7. Balsam of Peru (myroxylon pereirae): A natural fragrance ingredient derived from tree resin used in perfumes and skin lotions. Who said "natural" was better?

8. Fragrance mix: Common fragrance allergens found in cosmetic products. Manufacturers in the US must list this on the ingredient statements.

9. Formaldehyde: A much maligned preservative. You might remember the smell of this stuff from high school biology class.

10. Quaternium 15: Another preservative used in some cosmetic products.

The study was done using a method called patch testing in which human volunteers allow researchers to stick patches of these chemicals on their bodies for hours and days on end. For this the volunteers usually get paid about $50 bucks (US). Some people will do anything for a buck. Of course, I've personally participated in these kinds of studies purely for the advancement of science.

We here at the Beauty Brains are willing to suffer for our craft.

Should You Worry About Pee In Your Make Up

Meagan Muses:
I love your site– it makes me feel smarter all the time. I've got a question about diazolidinyl urea. I see it on labels for lotions and cleansers all the time. Doesn't urea come from urine? That seems disgusting to me. What's the story?

The Right Kidney, uh, Right Brain, Replies:
You're sort of right Meagan, but not really.

What is urea

Let's start by explaining that "diazolidinyl urea" is a preservative and it's used in many cosmetics to keep microscopic bugs from spoiling the products you bought with your hard earned money. It so happens that urea is one of the compounds used to make this ingredient. In addition, urea is also used in some creams and lotions as a moisturizer. So urea is used in cosmetics, but does urea really come from urine?

What is urine

Well, urine DOES contain urea. That's because urea excretion is just one of the ways your body gets rid of the excess nitrogen waste material that it generates. Different animals process this waste in different ways: Aquatic organisms excrete it in the form of ammonia. Reptiles and birds excrete it in the form of uric acid. And we humans excrete it in the form of urea.

Does urea come from urine

But fret not - the source of the urea used to make cosmetic ingredients is not someone's bladder. Industrial urea is synthetically made in large chemical reactors which are rarely, if ever, peed into. As a matter of fact, urea was the FIRST organic chemical ever to be synthetically created from inorganic starting materials. Back in 1828 chemist Friedrich Woehler reacted potassium cyanate with ammonium sulfate to create urea! Ah, there's nothing quite like a piece of chemical trivia like that to put a sparkle in my eye!

So in summary, the basic message of today's post is that we should all get down on our knees right now and thank Dr. Woehler for inventing urea so we don't have to worry about whether or not some stranger had to pee in our Clinique lotion in order to stop bacteria from growing in it.

Or something like that.

The Perils Of Parabens

Snapdragon77 asked:
Everyone is afraid of PARABENS! The product line that I use (Bioelements) lists methyl-paraben and propylparaben as the last ingredients, and I know that they are preservatives, but what do I tell a frightened clientele who have just heard "Parabens=Bad!"

The Left Brain Responds:
What are parabens?
Parabens are preservatives used in nearly every kind of cosmetic. They are put in formulas in small amounts to prevent the growth of disease-causing microbes. Without preservatives, cosmetics would be much more dangerous to use. They have been used in cosmetics for at least 20 years and are quite effective at killing microbes.

It's not surprising that parabens raise so many questions. Stories about these ingredients and the perils of using products that contain them are found everywhere on the net. A quick google search of parabens and cancer results in over 300,000 hits! Some sites extol the evils of parabens while others state a much different, less alarming position. So who should you believe?

Here's what the FDA has to say about the subject. Their position is best summed up in the following quote, "FDA believes that at the present time there is no reason for consumers to be concerned about the use of cosmetics containing parabens." But they are still looking at data.

And the primary governmental agency (in the United States) that receives money to research such questions, the National Institute for Health, has this position paper. Basically, researchers at the National Cancer Institute (NCI) are not aware of any conclusive evidence linking the use of underarm antiperspirants or deodorants and the subsequent development of breast cancer.

Why do people think parabens are bad?

So where did the furor about parabens and cancer come from? In 2004, Dr Philippa Darbre at the University of Reading published a study in the Journal of Applied Toxicology that said his group tested 20 different human breast tumors and found parabens in all of them. Neither he nor anyone else could explain how they got there or why they were there. They also couldn't say whether normal tissue had parabens. This raised the possibility that the parabens could have something to do with the cancer, but no one could explain what was going on. And since then, there still hasn't been an explanation. This doesn't mean parabens have anything to do with cancer. We just can't say they don't.

So, what do we think?

Here at the Beauty Brains, we have to side with the majority of the scientific research. Namely, at the moment there's no significant reason to be concerned. The notion that parabens are a major cause of breast cancer is just not true! It's possible that they might play a role in breast cancer but there is no conclusive evidence that supports this idea. No matter how bad parabens are, microbes are much worse.

Many cosmetic industry suppliers are offering alternatives to parabens. Privately, these companies acknowledge that parabens are more effective. They also do not believe there are any real safety issues, but it is an opportunity to create new products so they are taking it. Unfortunately, every other effective preservative such as DMDM Hydantoin (a formaldehyde releasing ingredient) or Kathon (synthetic) have potential safety issues. And suggested alternatives like grapefruit seed extract · phenoxyethanol · potassium sorbate · sorbic acid · tocopherol (vitamin E) · vitamin A (retinyl) · vitamin C (ascorbic acid) don't really work too well. The available preservatives aren't perfect, but they are the best there is. And they are certainly better than using nothing. Bacteria, yeast, and mold could really kill you!

The Beauty Brains bottom line.
Preservative alarmists may have a point and the industry is constantly on the lookout for new, effective ingredients. They just haven't found any. But the risk posed from these ingredients is so small that it's not worth worrying about. There are much more critical things you can do to avoid cancer like not smoking, avoiding excessive sun exposure, exercising regularly and eating a well-balanced, low fat diet. Don't waste your energy fretting about the preservatives in your cosmetics.

Top 5 Myths About Mineral Oil Part 1

We often see the advice that people should avoid mineral oil at all costs. This idea is propogated by numerous "natural" companies. Well, this advice is just bogus. It's not based on any scientific studies. Mineral oil is a perfectly fine ingredient and has been used in cosmetics for over 100 years.

Here are the top 5 Myths that companies tell people to make them afraid of mineral oil. In part 2 we look at why "natural" companies would be trying to scare you.

1. Mineral oil is contaminated with carcinogens
While it's true that some petroleum derivatives contain carcinogenic materials (like some polycyclic aromatic compounds) the mineral oil that is used in the cosmetic and pharmaceutical industry is highly refined and purified. It's purity is even regulated by the US FDA and other international regulatory

agencies. There is absolutely no evidence that cosmetic grade mineral oil causes cancer. And there has been plenty of testing done to ensure that fact. We could find no published reports in any of the dermatological or medical journals indicating a link between mineral oil and any forms of cancer.

2. Mineral oil dries the skin and causes premature aging
Mineral oil works as a barrier between the skin and the air. It acts as an occlusive agent which prevents water from naturally leaving your body through your skin. It will not dry out your skin or cause premature aging. Quite the contrary. It will provide moisturization.

3. Mineral oil robs the skin of vitamins
Since many vitamins are oil based, people assume that mineral oil will pull them out of your skin. There is no legitimate scientific evidence that this is true. Mineral oil has no effect on the vitamin levels in your skin.

4. Mineral oil prevents absorption of collagen from collagen moisturizers
Collagen in your skin lotions and moisturizers is too big to actually penetrate your skin. Therefore, mineral oil will have no effect on whether the collagen gets absorbed or not.

5. Mineral oil causes acne
In some people, mineral oil can exaserbate acne problems. However, most people will not experience any problems.

So, if it is not for safety concerns, why would companies be telling you to avoid mineral oil? We'll look at that in part 2 of our series.

The Beauty Brains bottom line
Mineral oil is NOT bad for you or your skin. It is one of the best ingredients available in skin lotions and moisturizers. It is also 100% natural taken directly out of our dear Mother Earth.

Myths About Mineral Oil Part 2

In part one of this series we looked at some of the things that are said about mineral oil and examined whether they were true or not. In part two we'll propose a few reasons why companies would try to propagate myths about mineral oil.

1. They want you to buy from them instead of the big manufacturers

This is the primary explanation for mineral oil bashing. Little companies have to find a way to convince consumers to use their products instead of the less expensive, name brands produced by large manufacturers. They can't possibly advertise as much as the big guys so they need other ways to motivate consumers. Spreading rumors, half truths, and lies about mineral oil (and a host of other ingredients) will scare a significant amount of people.

And most people don't have the time or scientific background to question what they hear. They'll just believe a myth about mineral oil causing cancer and avoid it at all costs. The lack of skepticism in our country is extremely troubling to this half of the Beauty Brains.

2. They need to have a reason why their products don't work as well

The truth is mineral oil is one of the best functioning skin care ingredients available. Every cosmetic chemist who reads studies published in the Journal of the Society of Cosmetic Chemists knows it. Other oils work too, but not as well as mineral oil.

When chemists are told they need to create a formula without mineral oil to satisfy a marketing story, they can't produce the best functioning product out there. It's a bit like trying to make omletes with egg beaters. Sure, it tastes like an omlete but it's not nearly as good as on made with real eggs. That's how it is with these "natural" type products.

3. They think natural things are inherently good

You find this notion throughout society but especially in the areas of cosmetics. In the US some people automatically believe that something taken directly from nature is better than something that is man-made or synthetic. Of course, there is no evidence supporting this notion and plenty of evidence to show that it is wrong. Natural is NOT necessarily better! Snake venom is natural. Cyanide is natural. Uranium is natural. Natural can be both good and bad. Similarly, synthetic things can be both good and bad.

The thing that is most amusing is that mineral oil is "natural". It is pulled right out of Mother Earth and purified for use in your favorite cosmetic. There is no synthetic process, just simple distillation of naturally occurring oil. Even an ingredient like Panthenol requires some chemical modification. Not mineral oil. Just natural purification.

4. They believe all of the myths about mineral oil

Despite the fact that there are some companies that are just trying to scare and lie to you, there are some people that honestly believe all they've read about the evils of mineral oil. And who could blame them? We all lead busy lives and when you hear bits of information that sound plausible, you don't have time to read the supporting research. Consequently, a manufacturer might believe they've found a much better product when they really haven't. People want to believe they can solve other people's problems. Even if their solution is based on a delusion.

The Beauty Brains bottom line

There are many reasons that myths about mineral oil continue. Chalk some up to naivete but others are downright fraud. You can believe whatever you want, just don't accept everything you hear about chemicals. You could be buying in to someone else's delusion. And that will cost you.

Should You Be Worried About Spermicide in Your Spa Cream?

Teresa has Trepidations:
I was shopping for high end spa products and noticed that their exfolliant cream contains Nonoxynol-9, a famously debated spermicide ingredient! I'm assuming it's not there to keep my freshly smoothed skin from becoming pregnant. So why is it in my creme and is there any downside to using it?

The Right Brain calms her down:
Take a deep breath Teresa, there's nothing to worry about.

Some creams contain detergents
Nonoxynol-9 (or N-9) is in your spa cream to help the dissolve the oil soluble ingredients in the cream base. That's because it's a surfactant (which is short for surface active agent) which is just a fancy way of saying it's a type of detergent. The cool thing is that N-9 is a nonionic surfactant which is a special type that doesn't create a lot of lather. Otherwise the spa cream would get all foamy when you rub it into your skin.

Detergents can be spermicidal
It just so happens that N-9's ability to dissolve oil into water has a very important side effect – it can also dissolve the acrosomal membranes of sperm, which stops the little guys from swimming. That's why it's used in many spermicidal creams, jellies, foams, gel, film, and suppositories. So, N-9 serves double duty: shy spa-cream emulsifier by day; sultry sperm-killer by night.

Finally, I feel compelled to point out that this discussion reminds me of the Seinfeld episode about being "sponge-worthy."

What You Should Know About Pregnancy And Cosmetics

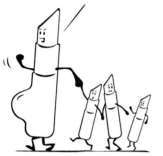

Oh, your father is getting snipped!!

Franca speaks frankly:
I've heard that you should avoid putting certain ingredients on your skin when you're pregnant. Are salicylic acid, self-tanners, and sunscreens safe to use whey you're expecting? Are there any other ingredients or skincare products pregnant women should avoid?

The Right Brain gestates this reply:
Experts agree that you should limit unnecessary drug exposure when you're pregnant. Here's what we found out from two expert sources: the American Pregnancy Association and American Academy of Dermatologists.

Five Facts About Pregnancy and Skin Care Ingredients
1. **Retin–A** (Isotretinoin) is a prescription acne medication that can cause cardiac problems in a fetus.

2. **Minoxidil** (aka Rogaine) the over-the-counter hair loss drug, is also known to contribute to birth defects.

3. **Fluconazole** is a topical antifungal drug that can also be teratogenic (causes birth defects).

4. **Sunscreens and Sunless Tanners** appear to be fine. There have been no reports of babies born with problems related to the mother's use of sunscreens. In fact, since UV radiation may cause folic acid deficiency, which can lead to neural tube defects like spina bifida, sunscreens could actually help!

5. **Salicylic acid facial products** are apparently low risk as well. But muscle creams containing a related compound (methyl salicylate) can be dangerous if overused, even if you're not pregnant.

The Beauty Brains bottom line
We hope this info is helpful but please be sure to check with your doctor to make sure you're doing everything right for your baby's health.

5 Ways Beauty Products Can Go Bad

Karen is quizzical:
Do beauty products have expiration dates hidden on the package? Whenever I see a great deal for an expensive beauty product on eBay or at a discount store like Marshalls, I wonder if the product has expired and is no longer as effective.

The Right Brain responds:
There's no way to tell if a cosmetic has expired just by looking at the package, but we can tell you what to look for when products go bad.

1. Changes in odor
Fragrances are made of dozens of different ingredients that can react with the rest of the product. It's not surprising then, that the fragrance is often the first thing to go bad. A little fragrance fading is totally normal, but if you detect a sour or rancid odor it may be a signal that something is seriously wrong.

2. Color shifting
The color of the product is very sensitive to light, so it's not unusual for cosmetics in clear packaging to experience a shift in shade. Slight color changes don't necessarily mean there's anything functionally wrong the product but you certainly don't want your red lipstick to become to orangey.

3. Change in texture
Changes in the consistency of a product may be subtle but significant. For example, if your skin lotion looks exceptionally thick or thin, or if it appears too grainy, this may be an early indicator of emulsion instability.

This means the oil and water soluble chemicals are separating. Not good!

4. Microbial contamination

If you see any black spots or fuzzy growth in your product, it could be contaminated with bacteria or fungus. Get rid of it immediately or you may be at risk for infection! And by the way, you should never dilute a product with water just so you can get the last little bit out of the bottle. Adding water can dilute the preservative system which can allow potentially dangerous bugs to grow.

5. Physical separation

If the product has separated into two layers it's gone bad. You can't always fix it by just remixing it. This is particularly true of cosmetics that have active ingredients like sunscreens and dandruff shampoos. Once the active drug ingredient has separated from the rest of the formula, it may not work properly anymore.

Do cosmetics have expiration dates?

In the United States cosmetic products are not required to have expiration dates. That's not really a bad thing because it's difficult, if not impossible, to really predict to the exact shelf life of any giving cosmetic products. (European products must be stamped with a Period After Opening date – we'll tell you about that another time.) The shelf life of any given product depends at least in part on how it's stored. Products can be stable for several years if they're kept away from light and heat, the two biggest enemies of cosmetics. But that same product can start to show fragrance degradation and color shift in a few weeks if exposed to sunlight and/or high temperatures.

The exceptions are over the counter drugs like dandruff shampoos, antiperspirants, fluoride toothpastes and acne products. The activity of drug ingredients in these products can be measured over time to estimate an expiration date. But it really doesn't work that way for non-drug products. But for the vast majority of cosmetic products it's a guessing game.

What about the secret code?

The bottom line is there's no way to tell just from looking at the package if the product is still good or not. But if you're really desperate there IS one thing you might try: look for the "secret" code that is the manufacturer's lot number. If you're shopping on Ebay and you see a product that you like, you can email them and ask if they can tell you the lot number off of the package. Then you could contact the maker of the product and ask them to tell you when it was made. That doesn't guarantee the product is good, but at least you can get an idea of it's age before you spend a lot of money on it.

Is Radiation From Cell Phones and Computers Bad For Your Skin

Bluz Cluz Smells A Bogus Claim:

Someone posted about this Clarins product which supposedly protects your skin from electromagnetic effects from cellphones and computers. Is this something that we should be concerned about? Seems like it's dressed-up toner. Would love your insight.

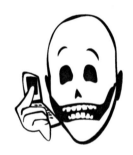

The Left Brain Laments Bad Science:

It's so refreshing to hear a little skepticism. This has got to be one of the most ridiculous new products I've heard about in a long time.

You are correct, this does appear to be a typical toner. While I couldn't find a complete ingredient list, I was amused to read about their "Magnetic Defense Complex with Thermus Chermophilus and Rhodiola Rosea, two powerful plant extracts which reinforce the skin's natural barrier and provide biological protection against electromagnetic waves." Puh-lease! This can't possibly work. To block electromagnetic fields you would need some kind of metal or insulator. This is just ridiculous.

The Beauty Brains bottom line

Even if these ingredients DID absorb EM radiation, you'd have to smear them ALL over your body before they would protect you. And finally, even if these ingredients DID work and even if you DID apply the product all over your body, there is absolutely no demonstrated negative effect on skin due to the electromagnetic fields created by cellphones or computers. So, we say save your money and don't sweat the "scary" electromagnetic fields.

Is Foreskin Good For Your Face?

Karen's curious:

There is a product called TNS Recovery Complex by Skin Medica that is made from (how can I say this tastefully?) a discarded piece of skin that some parents opt to have removed from their newborn baby boys before they leave the hospital. My dermatologist recommends and sells it. It has also been talked about enthusiastically on Oprah. Does this product really live up to the hype as an anti-aging, anti-wrinkle cream? It is VERY expensive!

The Left Brain replies:

According to the Skin Medica website, TNS contains an ingredient called NouriCel-MD which is their tradename for a combination of Natural Growth Factors, matrix proteins, and soluble collagen. You've seen proteins and collagen before but you may not know that Natural Growth Factors are a new category of compounds that act as chemical messengers to turn on and off a variety of cellular activities.

Do Natural Growth Factors work?

Theoretically, these compounds could have anti-aging properties when used in cosmetics. However, although products like TNS do contain growth factors, it looks like this technology is still in the experimental stages. According to Dr. Farris of the American Academy of Dermatologists "A multi-center double-blinded clinical study is currently underway to assess the anti-aging effects of human growth factors, and I expect that we'll be hearing a lot about their potential in medical applications in the coming years." Until we see study results to the contrary, we assume this product is more marketing hype than scientific breakthrough.

Show me the foreskin
But where did the notion that TNS contains foreskin come from? As the AAD article points out, growth factors can be extracted from plants, cultured epidermal cells, placental cells, and human foreskins. Ah ha! Since growth factors CAN be derived from foreskin (as well as other sources) and since Skin Medica uses growth factors in their TNS product, you can see how someone could jump to the conclusion that TNS contains actual human foreskin.

In fact, according to Skin Medica, their Nouricel-MD ingredient was developed by a San Diego-based biotechnology company that patented a process for growing cell banks. So, until Skin Medica announces that their secret ingredient is really based on infant penile sheaths, our guess is that this is just another internet rumor. (Note to Skin Medica, we've already written your next ad slogan: Foreskin - For Skin!)

Update on 4/21/07: *We did find a reference to an Oprah show where it was announced that this product contains an ingredient "engineered" from human foreskin cells. We're looking into this to find out exactly what that means. Stay tuned...*

Update on 4/22/07: *Dr. Rob Oliver, a Friend of the Brains and author of the Plastic Surgery 101 blog, says it's possible that TNS contains an ingredient that is DERIVED from foreskin cells. That doesn't mean that Skin Medica is chopping up foreskins and putting them in their product. You can read his remarks in the comment section on the blog. Thanks Dr. Rob!*

4 Ways To Tell If Your Cosmetic Has Expired

Gilda's guilty of using old product:
I have a Matrix Sleek Look shampoo and conditioner I bought 3 years ago, Can I use it? Is it effective?

The Right Brain reassures her:
Three years for a shampoo or conditioner is not out of the question, so your Matrix might be fine. But what about cosmetic products in general? if you're really worried that your product being past it's peak, ask yourself the following questions. If the answer to any of these is YES, then you might want to splurge on a replacement.

1. Does it fail the See and Sniff test?
Most cosmetics are designed to last a couple of years. A shampoo or conditioner like Matrix will probably still be fine. But before you use an old product, squeeze a little bit out and look at it and sniff it. Does it still smell okay? Maybe the fragrance just faded a bit. But if any of the ingredients have gone rancid or if there's microbial growth, you'll smell an off odor. Also look for junk growing in the product like mold or fungus. If you see or smell anything funky, don't use it! Likewise, if the product changed consistency and has become way too thick or way too thin, that's a signal that something changed. And not for the better!

2. Is it past the expiration date?
Ok, this one's tricky because most products don't HAVE an expiration date. Over The Counter Drug products do, but most regular cosmetics won't.

If you don't see an expiration date but you do see another string of numeric or alphanumeric code on the bottle, it's probably the lot code. The lot code tells the company when (and even where) the product was made. It's meant to help the company track the product so if you call them, they can tell you when the product was made and they should be able to recommend how long you can keep it before it expires.

By the way, in Europe, a new law requires a PAO (Period After Opening symbol) on the package. It looks like a little jar with a number on it and it tells you how many months the product is good for after you first start using it. You'll also see this symbol on some US products.

3. Was it stored improperly?

Some products are sensitive to heat, cold, and light. For example, we recently wrote about Babor's Intelli-zyme product that contains enzymes. Enzymes are notoriously unstable at high temperatures. Products like this can easily go bad from heat exposure. On the other hand, emulsion products, like skin lotions, can crystallize, thicken, or turn to mush if they're frozen. There's no way to know what happened to a product BEFORE you bought it, but you can take care to store it properly once you get it home. Don't leave products in the trunk of your car on a hot day or a cold day.

Then of course there's the condition of the package. Was it stored in a tightly sealed opaque bottle? Then there's less chance that light or air could have caused any problems. But if the lid is loose and it's in a clear glass bottle that sat in the window for 3 months, forget it!

4. Does it contain any "special" ingredients that are fragile?

If it's a regular product, like the Matrix example mentioned above, you probably don't have much to work about. But some active ingredients are a bit finicky, and those products can expire much sooner. Products like Babor's Intelli-zyme and even sunscreens are much more delicate. Click here if you want to read our previous post about how to tell if your sunscreen's gone bad.

Myths About Antiperspirants and Breast Cancer

Janessa, Sally, and several others in The Beauty Brains community have asked about the health risks associated with using antiperspirants. While we share your concerns, it turns out that most of those rumors are just that: rumors. How do we know that? Because we trust the research done by the experts in the medical field. So, fresh from the American Cancer Society's website, we present the true story:

The Top 5 Myths About Antiperspirants
1. Antiperspirants increase a person's risk of developing breast cancer.
2. Applying antiperspirant after shaving allows chemicals to enter the body from the armpit area and increase breast cancer risk.
3. Parabens in antiperspirants cause disease.
4. Antiperspirants keep a person from sweating cancer-causing toxins out through their underarm lymph nodes, resulting in accumulation of these toxins in breast tissue.
5. Men are less likely to get breast cancer because antiperspirant gets caught in the underarm hair and is not absorbed by their skin.

Click through to the ACS site for the full explanation on why these myths are false. And don't believe everything you read on the internet unless the information can be traced to a credible source. That's one of the basic beliefs of The Beauty Brains.

Will Covering Your Body With Antiperspirant Suffocate You?

Jessica is perspicacious about perspiration:
Is there any danger in applying antiperspirant on large areas of the body? For example, on the under arms, back, hairline etc.?

The Right Brain responds with dry wit:
Jess, sounds like you might have a case of hyperhydrosis, a condition that causes your sweat glands to kick into overdrive. So before we talk about antiperspirants, let's explain the source of sweat.

Where does sweat come from?

There two types of sweat glands on your body: eccrine glands and apocrine. Eccrine glands are found all over your body but most concentrated on the palms of hands, soles of feet, and the forehead. These glands produce sweat that is water and some salts and they are important in regulating body temperature. Sweat from eccrine glands doesn't cause body odor.

Apocrine glands are not as widespread. They are always associated with hair follicles so they show up wherever there is body hair, like in your arm pits and…uh…other areas. Apocrine glands produce a milky sweat that contains fatty materials. Bacteria that feed on these fatty materials create the unique smell of sweat.

How do antiperspirants stop sweating?

The active ingredient in antiperspirants are aluminum salts. Aluminum ions from these salts are absorbed by the cells that line the eccrine gland ducts. When water mixes with the salt, the cells swell up and form a plug that closes the gland so more sweat can't get out. A typical antiperspirant can decrease your sweat by at least 20 percent. Extra strength products, available by prescription, are even more effective. (Want to learn more? Read our post on how to avoid antiperspirant irritation.)

Can you use antiperspirant all over your body?

This question reminds us of the story of the actress in the James Bond film Goldfinger who supposedly died from asphyxiation after being covered with gold paint. Fortunately, this story turns out to be an urban myth – your body doesn't "breath" through your skin so you can't really suffocate. However, eccrine glands do help control body temperature and if you blocked all your sweat glands, your body would be in danger of over heating.

We couldn't find any medical references that explained exactly how much antiperspirant it takes to really be dangerous. The best we could come up with is this reference from Unilever (makers of Degree) that warns antiperspirants are "…really only designed for reducing underarm sweat and they should never be sprayed all over your body as you may overheat if too many sweat glands are blocked."

It seems like a reasonable caution to us but it's not a very satisfying answer if you're drenched in sweat. If hyperhydrosis is really a problem for you, we'd suggest checking with your doctor about using prescription strength antiperspirants or even more drastic measures like electrical treatments or Botox injections that can temporarily stun the sweat glands.

3 Reasons Why It's Ok To Have Toxins in Cosmetics

Lin longs to learn about Ammonium Hydroxide:
I've noticed it in several skincare products (like Neostrata AHA gel) and I'm worried because I read on a medical website that Ammonium hydroxide is a toxin and is found in many industrial products and cleaners such as flooring strippers, brick cleaners, and cements. And worst of all they warn you not to get it on your skin or in your eyes. Why is this toxic chemical in cosmetics?

The Right Brain lends a hand:
Thanks, Lin. Consumers should be asking questions like this to find out if their cosmetics are safe. But believe it or not, a lot of cosmetic (and food products!) contain ingredients that can be harmful at high concentrations. It's actually perfectly safe to use ingredients like this as long as they're formulated properly. Here are three reasons occasions that it's ok to have toxic chemicals in cosmetics.

1. Present at low levels
The ingredient can be added to the formula at such a low level that it has no negative effect whatsoever. Some preservatives are irritating when applied

directly to the skin. But when used at very low levels in a product they are much more easily tolerated by most people.

2. Used up in a reaction
The ingredient can be used up or reacted so it's not actually present in the finished product in a harmful form. Ammonium hydroxide is a good example of this type: it reacts with acidic materials in the formula and is neutralized to form a safe salt.

3. It's not abused
The ingredient can be dangerous if abused, but is safe if used properly. For example, a hair relaxer is very dangerous if you swallow it or get it in your eye. But when you use this toxic product properly, there's usually no problem. (Although some people do find relaxers irritating.)

The Beauty Brains bottom line
Obviously, we're being a little tongue-in-cheek here. We're not saying that ALL toxic ingredients should be treated as safe. We're just saying that you shouldn't over react to something you read on website when the information is provided out of context. Ammonium hydroxide is not something you have to worry about in your skin lotion.

Are Natural Products Better Than Processed?
The Parasites Think So

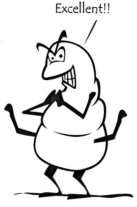

Excellent!!

This press release from the FDA about Cryptosporidium parasites in Baby's Bliss Gripe Water reminded me of the reasons to stay away from any herbal supplement and to be skeptical of any company that touts "natural" as a reason to buy. People who have dutifully given Baby's Bliss Gripe Water to their infants now have the added benefit of knowing they may have given them a parasite too. If you are one of those parents who have a bottle with code 26952V and an expiration date of 10/08, return the product immediately.

Herbal Supplement Outrage
And then ask yourself why are you giving an unregulated, unnecessary herbal supplement to a child? As we previously discussed, Herbal Supplement Companies Are Not Regulated! And the FDA does not have enough resources to test every supplement product put on the market. You have no way to know whether the product is safe or not. Unlike food manufacturers, there is no law that requires independent testing of the products made and sold by herbal supplement manufacturers. It's complete nonsense. These supplements can have real health effects and it's only through shear luck that problems are discovered. Why is it that the FDA had to find the parasite when the company MOM Enterprises, Inc. couldn't? Clearly something is messed up.

The Nonsense of Natural Products
I see that MOM Enterprises also sells a line of personal care products. Hopefully, they don't rely on the 'naturalness' of their raw materials and they treat them to remove disease causing parasites, bacteria and viruses. These are the kinds of things that preservatives are designed to kill. Yes, preservatives protect us from the evil things found in Natural Products.

It is interesting that Baby's Bliss has a Diaper Cream they claim to be "100% natural". Then they show in their list of ingredients...

- Caprylic/Capric Triglyceride
- Cetearyl Olivate (and) Sorbitan Olivate
- Cetyl Alcohol
- Stearic Acid
- Glycine
- Zinc Oxide
- Dimethicone
- Fragrance

Where in nature can you find Dimethicone? I know it's derived from sand but you have to go through a lot of chemical processing to make Dimethicone. This product isn't 100% Natural. It's processed. And that's a good thing. Processed products are safer products!

The Beauty Brains bottom line:
When you don't process and chemically alter natural things you end up with PARASITES or bacteria or other disease causing microbes. That's not something you want.

And if you are in the United States and you're giving herbal supplements to your children, you're taking a huge risk! The products are unregulated and in this Beauty Brain's opinion, unsafe for children.

Appendix A
Beauty Brains Quiz

A popular feature of the Beauty Brains blog is our weekly beauty science or BS quiz. We find 3 science stories that are true and make one up. You have to figure out which one is the fake. Good luck.

1. Which of these statements about men and women's skin is NOT TRUE?
   A. Coffee can improve a man's skin, but not a woman's.
   B. A woman's skin ages faster than a man's.
   C. A man's skin is more prone to skin cancer than a woman's.
   D. A man's skin is 50% thicker than a woman's
   E. A woman's skin is less oily than a man's.

2. Which one of the skin stories below is the fake one?
   A. Drinking tea may protect your skin
   B. Smearing black raspberries on your skin may protect it
   C. Oil used to cook French Fries may repair damaged skin
   D. Playing a musical instrument may be good for your skin

3. Which one of the hair stories below is the fake one?
   A. Hair can expose eating disorders
   B. Tea drinking can speed hair growth
   C. Oil spills can be cleaned with hair
   D. Lizards use hair to stick to surfaces

4. Which one of the skin stories below is fake?
   A. Your skin color may be influenced by what your grandmother ate
   B. Melanin can make you more susceptible to skin cancer
   C. Regular running makes you more prone to skin cancer.
   D. High stress can increase acne severity

5. Which one of the following beauty devices are not really for sale?
   A. Wand that shoots oxygen into your skin to smooth and tone
   B. Hand held laser that makes your hair grow
   C. Electronic headband that relaxes muscles to remove wrinkles
   D. Ceramic unipolar magnet that controls acne

6. Which one of the beauty research studies below is made up?
   A. Rich people are more prone to skin cancer.
   B. Prolonged use of muscle pain cream can kill you.
   C. You can become addicted to tanning.
   D. Your skin is home to over 182 species of mites.

7. Which one of the beauty stories below is fake?
   A. Nanotechnology was used for hair dyes 2000 years ago
   B. Women dress better when they're less fertile
   C. Hypnosis can help cure skin disorders
   D. Bull semen is used to increase hair shine

8. Which one of the following stories about the beauty industry are fake?
    A. People with facial acne are more likely to get back acne
    B. PETA kills thousands of animals each year
    C. Strippers taking birth control pills earn less money
    D. Temporary black henna dyes can cause permanent scarring

9. Which one of the following stories about the beauty industry are fake?
    A. Some people hear colors and see sounds.
    B. Men prefer reddish colors more than women.
    C. Excessive vitamin use can lead to heart disease.
    D. Flesh-eating fish are used to exfolliate skin.

10. What odor has been scientifically proven to turn men on the most?
    A. Buttered Popcorn
    B. Black Licorice and Cola
    C. Pumpkin Pie and Lavender
    D. Orange

Answers:

10. C   To see a complete explanation of all the Beauty Brains quiz
9. B   questions, please visit the website at the following address.
8. A
7. B   http://www.thebeautybrains.com/quiz
6. D
5. D
4. C
3. B
2. D
1. D

Appendix B
Useful Resources

It is our hope that reading the Beauty Brains will make everyone a smarter consumer who makes informed decisions when purchasing beauty products.

While you can learn something new every day on the Beauty Brains blog, there are a number of other great resources for finding more beauty product information and advice.

Consumer Reports
(www.consumerreports.org/cro/health-fittness/beauty-personal-care)
This is the online version of the magazine. It features information about a variety of beauty and personal care products including reserached reports on sunscreens, wrinkle creams, anti-aging products and more. They have good information and get many things right.

The Cosmetics Cop
(www.cosmeticscop.com)

Paula Begoun started her career as make-up artist, moved to television as a beauty reporter and finally became the Cosmetics Cop authoring several best selling books about the beauty industry such as Don't Go to the Cosmetics Counter Without Me and The Beauty Bible. Her website and books feature reviews of thousands of cosmetics and personal care products. She does an excellent job of reviewing both the products and some of the science behind them.

Quack Watch
(http://quackwatch.com)

While this site is dedicated to primarily health related topics, it provides an excellent foundation for critical thinking and evaluation of the claims, demos and bunk used to sell cosmetics and beauty products. You can find a number of articles about how to protect yourself from quackery you'll see all around you.

U.S. Food and Drug Administration
(www.cfsan.fda.gov/~dms/cos-toc.html)

Contrary to what some sources claim, the FDA does provide regulatory guidelines for the cosmetic industry. At this website you can find information about a number of cosmetic issues such as ingredient and product descriptions, labeling requirements, recall information and even a quiz to test how smart you are about cosmetics.

Personal Care Products Council - Cosmetics Info
(www.cosmeticsinfo.org)

This website is run by the cosmetic industry oversite council who is responsible for ensuring that cosmetics in the U.S. comply with accepted standards. They provide good scientific information, but it is not completely unbiased since it's run by cosmetic manufacturers.

American Academy of Dermatology
(www.aad.org)
This site provides a wealth of free information regarding nearly every type of skin condition known. You can find advice for how to deal with acne, eczema, psoriasis and other common skin problems. It also gives great information for finding a dermatologist in your area.

Society of Cosmetic Chemists
(www.scconline.org/website/news/ask_the_expert.shtml)
If you want to know more about cosmetics and you're not getting a response quick enough from the Beauty Brains (we get swamped with questions) try the SCC's Ask the Expert page. Simply fill out their form and send in your question. It will be answered by a member of the Society of Cosmetic Chemists. Of course, it won't be as clever as the Beauty Brains' response, but you'll get good information.

The Demon-Haunted World - Science as a Candel in the Dark
BY CARL SAGAN
Sagan is a wonderful writer and this book is one of his best works. In it he explains how science can be used to understand the world better. Of particular interest to skeptical beauty afficionados is Chapter 12 in which he provides a "balony detection kit" for determining if something is science or fiction.

Appendix C
Ingredient Lists

Perhaps the most important skill you can have when evaluating cosmetics is reading the ingredient list. In the cosmetic business it's called an LOI or List of Ingredients. Here is how you read them, what they mean, and where you can find more information.

In the United States, cosmetic manufacturers are compelled by the governing industry trade organization known as the Personal Care Products Council (formerly the Cosmetic, Toiletry and Fragrance Association) to include a list of ingredients on their labels. They maintain a book known as the International Cosmetic Ingredient Dictionary and Handbook which the names of nearly all the ingredients used in cosmetic products worldwide. It's quite a tome that makes groovy bedtime reading.

Why have the labels?

The labels are required because the industry wants consumers to know exactly what chemicals they are putting on their bodies. This will allow you to make choices as to what chemicals you want to be exposed to.

Of course, that assumes you know what any of the chemicals are, which for most consumers is not the case. Fortunately, with the internet you can simply look up chemical names using a search engine to get more information about the compounds. Be careful however, there are plenty of sites loaded with misinformation about perfectly safe chemicals. Compounds like propylene glycol, mineral oil, and sodium lauryl sulfate have been slandered by biased sources all over the internet. Read all things on the internet with a skeptical eye. We reject gurus and encourage everyone to become their own experts.

What does the label mean?

When properly written, the labels can provide you with a lot of useful information. In the United States, any chemical above 1% by weight in the formula is required to be listed in order of concentration. Below 1% the order can be anything they like. Typically, preservatives, fragrances, and colors are listed at the end. Let's look at an example of a skin moisturizer.

Ingredients: Water, Glycerin, Cetearyl Alcohol, Petrolatum, Mineral Oil, Ceteareth 20, Dimethicone, Glyceryl Dilaurate, Erythrulose, Persea Gratissima Fruit Extract (Avocado), Avena Sativa Meal Extract (Oat), Simmondsia Chinensis Seed Extract (Jojoba), Calendula Officinalis Flower Extract, Olea Europaea Fruit Oil (Olive), Tocopherol, Cyclopentasiloxane, Stearic Acid, Acrylates/C10 Alkyl Acrylate Crosspolymer, Methylparaben, Propylparaben, Citric Acid, Disodium EDTA, Sodium Hydroxide, DMDM Hydantoin, BHT, Fragrance, Caramel, Titanium Dioxide, Mica, Dihydroxyacetone

The first ingredient is water which means this formula is mostly water. Based on this Brain's knowledge of lotions, it is about 80% water. Glycerin is the next most abundant ingredient probably in there at about 5%. The next few ingredients are anywhere from 1-3%. Look at other skin lotions. I bet you find many of the same ingredients listed in the first line.

Now, when you get to a "natural" sounding ingredient like Persea Gratissima Fruit Extract you know you've dropped below the magic 1% level. This is where manufacturers can start to make things look different. Generally, natural ingredients are so expensive and less effective that only a very small amount is in there.

Most manufacturers like to put lots of these "feature" ingredients in the formula just so they have something to talk about and to show their formula are different. The truth is the real functional work of the product is done by the ingredients above this 1% line. This isn't strictly true as there are many ingredients that give quite good benefits below the 1% level, but generally it's true. The more abundant a material, the more function it will have.

Ingredient lists are included on your cosmetics to give you useful information about the products you use everyday. They are put together following specific rules and if you know these, you can learn a lot about a product. The next time you're thinking of spending $25 on that upscale hair conditioner, compare the ingredient list to the $3 bottle. You might be surprised by the striking similarities. And if the chemicals are the same, you can bet they'll work similiarly.

About the Authors

The Beauty Brains is written by a group of real cosmetic scientists with over 40 years of combined experience in the beauty industry. The questions contained in this book are from actual readers of the Beauty Brains blog. If you have beauty questions that were not answered in this book, please visit the blog and

Ask the Brains!

http://www.thebeautybrains.com

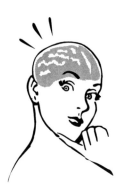

Printed in the United States
128644LV00005B/90/P